THE WHICH? GUIDE TO
COMPLEMENTARY MEDICINE

About the author

BARBARA ROWLANDS is a freelance writer specialising in
health issues. She contributes regularly to consumer and specialist
publications, as well as national newspapers. She is an editorial
consultant, a lecturer in journalism and a member of the Medical
Journalists' Association and the Guild of Health Writers.

Acknowledgements

THE AUTHOR and publishers would like to thank all the com-
plementary practitioners, doctors and researchers who were gen-
erous with their time, especially Dr Thurstan Brewin, Professor
Edzard Ernst, Dr Julian Kenyon, Dr George Lewith, Dr Virginia
Murray, Dr David Peters, Debbie Shaw, Dr Alan Watkins and Dr
Adrian White. The Research Council for Complementary
Medicine provided some of the information in the book.

We are indebted to the following people for their comments: Dr
Julian Greaves, Kevin Grealis and Gary Allison (Chapter 5), Dr
Colin Lewis and John Parkinson (acupuncture), David Howlett
(Alexander technique), Teddy Fearnhamm and Robert Tisserand
(aromatherapy), Dr. N. S. Moorthy (ayurvedic medicine), Ken
Lloyd (Chinese herbal medicine), Sue Cartlidge and Chris Turner
(chiropractic), Dr Milo Siewert (colonic hydrotherapy), Pauline
Wills (colour therapy), Stefan Ball (flower remedies), Dr Daniel
Benor and Commander David Repard (healing), Michael
McIntyre and Dr Simon Mills (herbal medicine), Dr Peter Fisher,
Stephen Gordon and Enid Segall (homeopathy), Dr Tom Bell
(hypnotherapy), Adam Jackson (iridology), Maggie La Tourelle
(kinesiology), Maria Mercati and Anne Tibbs (massage therapy), F.
Whiting, Vishvapani and Dr Michael West (meditation), Gaston
Saint-Pierre (metamorphic technique), Roger Newman Turner
(naturopathy), Brian Daniels (osteopathy), Angela Hope-Murray
and Hazel Goodwin (reflexology), Jenny Crewdson (rolfing),
Nicola Pooley (shiatsu) and Ghislaine Picchio (t'ai chi).

Thanks are also due to Helen Barnett, Pamela Baxter, David
Dickinson, John Francis and David Rodwell at Consumers'
Association.

THE WHICH? GUIDE TO
COMPLEMENTARY MEDICINE

BARBARA ROWLANDS

CONSUMERS' ASSOCIATION

Which? Books are commissioned and researched by
Consumers' Association and published by
Which? Ltd, 2 Marylebone Road, London NW1 4DF

Distributed by The Penguin Group:
Penguin Books Ltd, 27 Wrights Lane, London W8 5TZ

First edition February 1997
Copyright © 1997 Which? Ltd

British Library Cataloguing in Publication Data
A catalogue record for this book is available from the British Library

ISBN 0 85202 634 X

For a full list of Which? books, please write to
Which? Books, Castlemead, Gascoyne Way, Hertford X, SG14 1LH.

Index by Marie Lorimer
Cover design by Ridgeway Associates
Cover photograph by Les Wies/Tony Stone Images
Illustrations by Andrew Bezear

Typeset by Saxon Graphics Ltd, Derby

Printed and bound by Firmin-Didot (France), Group Herissey,
No d'impression: 37058

CONTENTS

Introduction   7

PART I   Complementary medicine and the consumer

1 Complementary therapies, their users and
   providers   13
2 Complementary medicine and the NHS   24
3 The scientific case for complementary medicine   29
4 Complementary medicine: the good, the bad
   and the unknown   35
5 Complementary medicine and the law   49

PART II   A-Z of complementary therapies

Acupuncture   71
Alexander technique   82
Aromatherapy   87
Art therapies   96
Ayurvedic medicine   101
Chinese herbal medicine   105
Chiropractic   113
Colonic hydrotherapy   120
Colour therapy   124
Crystal and gem healing   129
Flower remedies   132
Healing   136
Herbal medicine   144
Homeopathy   152
Hypnotherapy   161
Iridology   169
Kinesiology   175

Massage therapy   180
Meditation   187
Metamorphic technique   193
Naturopathy   197
Osteopathy   204
Radiesthesia and radionics   210
Reflexology   215
Rolfing   222
Shiatsu   226
T'ai chi   230
Yoga   233

Appendix: survey results   239
Glossary   245
Addresses   247
Bibliography   253
Index   261
Reader's report form   266

INTRODUCTION

WITH THE number of visits to complementary therapists running at over 4 million and the number of therapists increasing at the rate of some 11 per cent a year in the UK, complementary medicine is booming. The very term 'complementary medicine' is an indication of how acceptable the diverse therapies covered by it have become: what was once considered the prerogative of cranks or people who had more money than sense came gradually to be called 'alternative' medicine because it was used in place of orthodox medicine. Now, in the '90s, some therapies are being used *in conjunction* with mainstream medicine.

The popularity of complementary medicine is not restricted to users of such therapies: studies have shown that three-quarters of GP fundholding practices would like to see complementary medicine available on the National Health Service; four out of ten GPs already offer their patients complementary therapies.

The reasons for the phenomenal growth in popularity and acceptance of complementary medicine are many (they are explored in the first chapter of this book). Primarily, complementary medicine appeals to people because it can (assuming a competent therapist) meet four of the patient's most important needs:

- a good relationship with the practitioner
- a sense of personal control
- an understandable explanation of the illness
- effective treatment.

In addition, disillusionment with orthodox medicine, and exposure to foreign – especially Eastern – cultures have contributed to people's willingness to try complementary therapies.

The increase in their use, particularly in the late 1980s and early 1990s, has also come about because the public is better informed; many more of us are aware that modern medicine has its limitations, especially for chronic conditions, and some of us are disappointed with the impersonal nature of the conventional doctor-patient relationship, so we are choosing to exercise consumer choice.

Complementary medicine in the strictest sense means those non-orthodox therapies which are used in conjunction with mainstream medicine: for example, while cancer patients are being treated with chemotherapy or radiotherapy they can also have massage or aromatherapy to help them manage the stress and discomfort; elderly people and those with mental and physical disabilities can gain a sense of peace and calm through touch therapies, such as *reiki* or reflexology, while taking their medication. The industry itself uses the term in a looser sense, to include therapies which lie outside mainstream medicine: the 'alternative' therapies, such as homeopathy and herbal medicine, which are used in place of (rather than alongside) orthodox treatment. However, the distinction between complementary and alternative therapies is becoming blurred. Most reputable complementary practitioners are keen to work alongside conventional doctors and would never advise patients to come off their medication. For the purposes of this book, the term 'complementary medicine' will be used in its wider sense.

Complementary medicine is a very broad church. There are well over a hundred therapies, headed up by what the British Medical Association calls the 'discrete clinical disciplines' – acupuncture, homeopathy, herbal medicine, osteopathy and chiropractic, which are the most commonly used therapies in the UK today. The range and diversity of complementary therapies are considerable. They include crystal therapy, flower remedies, colour therapy, sound healing and colonic hydrotherapy. Some, such as traditional Chinese medicine, are thousands of years old; others, such as rolfing and the Alexander technique, have been in existence for less than a century. Some have been subjects of extensive scientific study, others have not. Some therapists are highly qualified and are wholly committed, others are not. Some therapies have regulatory bodies or well-established organisations to which they can be affiliated, others are run by one person. Some are highly successful businesses, turning over millions of pounds a year. Some of the regulatory bodies have thousands of practitioners on their books, while therapists who practise some of the more esoteric techniques can be thin on the ground.

This book offers an introduction to a range of therapies, some of them well established, widely respected and accorded a high level of credibility. Several minor therapies have also been included, because people are curious about what they are and how they are supposed to work: we offer brief accounts of some of these, if only to warn readers off wasting their time and money on them.

Certain therapies have been excluded. Traditional remedies, or 'folk medicine', have been left out because, while they might fall within the definition of a non-orthodox or complementary therapy, there are few practitioners and no umbrella organisation. The strength of folk medicine lies in the fact that it is easy for the lay person to administer – it is often something you do to yourself, based on 'old wives' tales' and information handed down from generation to generation. Many of these ancient cures work very well, such as the cooling effect of dock leaves on a nettle sting, and orthodox medicine has little hesitation in taking them on board.

Counselling has also been omitted, mainly because it is now such an accepted part of orthodox medicine, especially in pre-operative situations and for very serious illnesses.

The therapies in this book have been examined, as far as possible, with a critical eye. Many of them have little science to back them up, but appear to work none the less. The book explains the advantages and disadvantages of each and points out the dangers (if any) as well as the benefits. Unlike books on complementary therapies written by people with a vested interest in putting over a particular view, this guide takes an independent look at the therapies with which most people are likely to come into contact so that they can make informed choices.

Rather unusually for what is such a fast-growing business, little research has been done into the usage of complementary medicine. An appendix at the back of the book summarises one of the few national studies to have been carried out recently: a survey of

Which? subscribers, published in November 1995. A report form has been included in the book so that readers can tell us about their own experiences of complementary therapies and whether they found them beneficial. It is hoped that in due course there will be sufficient data for the findings to be published in *Health Which?* magazine.

Most complementary practitioners are well aware that they still have to prove to the world at large that their therapies work. They are now beginning to do so, with an ever-increasing body of scientific evidence to back up their claims. Such research is to be welcomed, as is the regulation of the industry, currently a slow and painful process undertaken by those within it. In the meantime, users of complementary medicine, most of whom are more confident of a successful outcome than the evidence currently warrants, are likely to carry on taking things on trust.

Note Addresses and telephone numbers for organisations marked with an asterisk (*) can be found in the address section at the back of the book.

'He/she': the pronoun 'he' has been used where to use both would impede the flow of the text.

PART I

COMPLEMENTARY MEDICINE AND THE CONSUMER

CHAPTER 1

COMPLEMENTARY THERAPIES, THEIR USERS AND PROVIDERS

COMPLEMENTARY medicine has not always been as popular in the UK as it is today. The reasons for the increase in acceptability and use of such therapies reveal a great deal about social trends in the second half of the twentieth century. This chapter explores the history of the growth in this field and looks at the kinds of people who are drawn to it. It also groups together the therapies covered in the book according to similarities in technique or origin and guides the reader through the tricky issues of what therapy to choose and how to find a reliable therapist.

The rise in popularity of complementary medicine

Even as recently as in the 1960s complementary medicine was a fringe interest in the UK; before the 1960s there was not even a general name by which these therapies were known.

People still had faith in mainstream medicine: most infectious diseases were under control, and improved hygiene and general living standards had cut down those illnesses resulting from poverty. Doctors were respected members of the post-war community, and they had the time to talk to and visit their patients. Old-fashioned practices, such as herbal medicine and homeopathy, were tolerated, partly, perhaps, because the royal family and upper classes favoured them, but therapies new to the West, such as acupuncture, were viewed as suspect.

A substantial shift in attitudes has taken place since then, corresponding with a growing disillusionment with conventional medicine and its approach to treatment. Despite the promises of the 1950s and '60s, medicine has failed to deal successfully with chronic ailments, such as irritable bowel syndrome and rheumatoid arthritis. The progress curve that began with the discovery of penicillin and insulin has not been maintained, and as yet we have no answers to the ailments of the late twentieth century such as stress-related disorders. In addition, cures for colds, 'flu and fatigue do not yet exist. Moreover, some of the side-effects resulting from taking certain orthodox medicines are irksome. These side-effects, real or imagined, are one of the main reasons why many people are turning to complementary medicine. In 1962 thalidomide, marketed in the UK under the brand name Distaval, was sold for two years to pregnant women to help quell morning sickness before it was realised that it caused babies to be born with malformations. The nature of the disabilities – babies were born without or with only rudimentary arms and legs – was shockingly severe. The public had to face up to the fact, as never before, that drugs could destroy as well as cure.

Another source of dissatisfaction has been the long waiting time for hospital treatment on the overstretched National Health Service. Many people who use chiropractic and osteopathy do so because the wait for orthodox treatment at a hospital is too long, given that they are suffering pain and discomfort.

It is not just the type of treatment by practitioners of conventional medicine that people are unhappy with; it is their approach as well. The NHS relied, and to a great extent still relies, on the compliant patient. When the GP does not have the answer, he or she will refer the patient to a hospital consultant who does. In general, the patient merely either complies or fails to comply.

But patients today are less accepting and more critical than they were in the 1950s. Most take the existence of the NHS for granted; although they value it, many choose complementary medicine to treat conditions which mainstream medicine manages poorly. Moreover, patients today are, by and large, much better informed than they used to be. Media reporting of medical advances and the availability of easily digestible accounts of diseases mean that patients often know a considerable amount about their condition.

Complementary medicine allows patients to take a more pro-active role in their treatment. This sense of control, a more personal relationship with the practitioner, the availability of a comprehensible explanation of their illness and the fact that complementary therapies often offer the hope of an effective treatment are the reasons people are drawn to complementary medicine.

Conventional doctors generally look for a cause of a specific ailment, such as a virus, and treat a patient for the particular condition. Most complementary therapists believe that disease is also triggered by environmental and emotional factors, which is why they tend to treat the person as a whole. The holistic approach, which takes emotional – and sometimes spiritual – health as well as physical condition into consideration, has found favour with many people (see Chapter 4).

Complementary medicine and the rest of the world

The popularity of complementary therapies is not confined to the UK; indeed, consumers in many other Western countries spend more than those in the UK on natural remedies and non-orthodox treatments.

A telephone survey in 1990 of adults in the United States found that a third of them had used some form of unconventional medicine in the previous year, spending a total of US$13.7 billion on the therapies, three-quarters of which (US$10.3 billion) was out-of-pocket. This is not far short of the total of US$12.8 billion spent out-of-pocket by all Americans on hospital treatment in the same period. Results from the survey suggest that Americans made 425 million visits to complementary practitioners compared with 388 million visits to primary-care physicians. This category includes GPs but not hospital doctors.

A survey published in March 1996 in Australia, the largest so far on the use of complementary medicine, revealed that one in five Australians regularly visits a complementary practitioner and that half of the population of the state of South Australia regularly turns to one. In 1993 Australians spent a total of A$930 million on visiting therapists and consuming complementary medicines. They spent roughly a third of that – A$360 million –

on conventional drugs. In New Zealand one in four GPs uses acupuncture.

In France the percentage of people who regularly visit a complementary therapist is 48, in Germany 46, in Belgium 31 and in the Netherlands 20. National preferences vary: for example, massage is very popular in Finland, the Dutch are keen on spiritual healers, and in France the most popular therapy is homeopathy – its use rose from 16 per cent of the population in 1982 to 36 per cent in 1992. In the UK just under one in ten people take herbal remedies, and the market for over-the-counter homeopathic medicines is growing by 20 per cent a year.

Who uses complementary medicine?

Few national surveys of the use of complementary medicine have been done in the UK. Consumers' Association conducted one in 1995, the results of which were published in the November 1995 issue of *Which?*. Of the nearly 9,000 subscribers to the magazine who responded, almost one in three had used complementary medicine at some time in their lives. Of those who had used it, one in five had done so during the preceding year. Women were more likely to have tried it than men: 40 per cent had done so, compared with 27 per cent of men. Interestingly, while 33 per cent of those aged above 35 had used complementary medicine, only 26 per cent of the below-35s had. More details of the findings are given in the appendix at the end of this book.

Other polls have shown that people living in the south of England visit more complementary practitioners than those living in the north and Scotland, and that complementary therapy is most popular in the west of England.

The Australian survey (see Complementary medicine and the rest of the world) found that most people who use complementary therapies are, not surprisingly, affluent.

The *Which?* study found that an increasing proportion of young, fit people are turning to complementary medicine. Although some people (41 per cent) turn to complementary medicine to alleviate long-term conditions, many use it to maintain and enhance their health – i.e. as preventive medicine. Another interesting fact is that many people (38 per cent in the survey) tend to use more than one complementary therapy, often at the same time.

There is also some evidence to support the popular belief that more women turn to the 'gentler' therapies such as aromatherapy or homeopathy than men do, even though they may use others such as osteopathy. This may tie in with the hypothesis that women are more likely to believe in the philosophy behind the therapies whereas men find it easier to credit something they can physically feel being done to them.

Types of complementary therapies

Complementary therapies generally fall into the following categories:

- touch therapies, such as massage, aromatherapy, metamorphic technique, reflexology and healing
- mind-body medicine, such as hypnotherapy, meditation and yoga
- manipulative and structural therapies, such as osteopathy, chiropractic and rolfing and yoga
- postural techniques, such as Alexander technique
- medicinal therapies, such as homeopathy, herbal medicine and flower remedies
- Oriental medicine, such as acupuncture and Chinese herbal medicine
- self-help, such as yoga, t'ai chi and meditation.

Some therapies fall into two categories. T'ai chi, for instance, is both an Oriental technique and a self-help therapy. Others have superficial similarities in philosophy, but are, in fact, quite distinct. Reflexology and metamorphic technique are both concerned with feet, but there the similarity ends. Acupuncture and yoga are both concerned with energy systems, but vary in the way that the energy is boosted. Some therapies, such as iridology, kinesiology and radionics, do not fit easily into any category.

Therapies differ markedly in the techniques they employ and their approach to the human body. Some involve direct intervention by way of pills or potions (herbalism) or the manipulation of the body (chiropractic); others, such as healing, involve just the laying-on of hands. A few, such as radionics, do not even require the patient's physical presence.

Some therapies adhere to the 'orthodox' view of the body, based on understanding accepted in the West, and enshrined in *Gray's Anatomy*; others, based on Eastern cultures, postulate that the body is laced with energy channels which can be manipulated and 'unblocked' (see Chapter 3).

The aims of the therapies and the ways in which they are practised also vary. Some techniques, such as kinesiology and iridology, are seldom used as stand-alone therapies but as tools by practitioners of other therapies. For example, a herbalist or a naturopath may use iridology to diagnose a patient's condition. While many therapies, such as Chinese herbal medicine, help cure specific conditions, others, such as aromatherapy, are used to promote a general sense of well-being. Therapies such as yoga and t'ai chi can be practised in groups or alone; others, such as osteopathy, involve being treated by the practitioner on a one-to-one basis.

Whether and how to opt for complementary therapy

Deciding whether to opt for therapy, and which one, can be daunting, especially given the number of therapies and the differences between them. Before considering the pros and cons of individual therapies, ask yourself why you want to use complementary medicine at all.

- Is making the decision to try complementary medicine valuable in itself? It is possible that it can make you feel that you are in control and are expressing a personal preference about how you want your body (and perhaps your mind) to be treated. Pressure from friends or relatives to try complementary medicine is not a good enough reason to do so.

- Are you consulting a therapist for the treatment of an existing ailment or for maintaining good health? If the former, think carefully about whether your expectations are realistic: are you looking to complementary medicine to cure a disorder or to alleviate the symptoms and help you live with it?

- Do you want to try complementary medicine because you are dissatisfied with conventional medicine? Do specific aspects of complementary medicine – for example, the holistic approach implicit in many therapies – attract you to it?

Whatever your reasons for trying complementary medicine, consult your GP before embarking upon any therapy and, equally important, ensure that you liaise with him or her throughout your treatment.

Many ailments and conditions can be cured or alleviated by more than one therapy: for instance, eczema can be treated by practitioners of ayurveda, Chinese herbal medicine, (Western) herbal medicine and homeopathy. Of those that are relevant for your needs, choose the one – or more – that appeals to you most in terms of its philosophy and technique. You may, for example, find the Chinese way of explaining ill-health in terms of blockages of *qi* (energy) a satisfactory one, but may have a fear of needles, which would rule out acupuncture. The likely cost and the availability in your area of a practitioner are also important considerations. Be prepared to commit yourself to a full course of treatment, and also to stop having it if, after a while, you feel it is not helpful.

It is, of course, possible – and common – to combine therapies. Indeed, many practitioners themselves use a range of therapies to treat a patient. A naturopath could use iridology as a diagnostic tool; a Chinese herbalist could (if appropriately qualified) incorporate acupuncture into the treatment; and an ayurvedic practitioner could use massage or yoga to treat you. If you choose to use different therapies at the same time ensure that your GP and the individual practitioners know about it.

How to find a reliable practitioner

Most people who visit a complementary practitioner are happy with their treatment. In a survey published in *Health Which?* in December 1995 only 85 out of a total of 2,635 who responded said that they had had a bad experience and that they wanted to complain. They fell into three categories: those who said there had been no change in their health; those who felt that the cost of the treatment was too high; and those who felt that they had suffered injury.

If you want to try complementary medicine, your best chance of being a satisfied customer is to find a good practitioner. This is not just a question of avoiding quacks; it is equally important to choose a practitioner you are comfortable with.

Personal recommendation is usually the best way of finding a reputable therapist, but not always. A friend or colleague may have built up a rapport with the therapist, but you may not be able to. It is still worth checking out the therapist's credentials. You can take advice from your GP, but he or she may be unenthusiastic about complementary therapies as a whole and, indeed, may be no better informed than you are. Your local natural healing centre will be a good source of the names of local practitioners and the staff will probably be able to suggest which therapy would suit you. Natural healing centres usually have several practitioners with different skills working there.

Do not look for therapists at natural healing fairs and festivals, or in advertisements displayed in libraries and newsagents, and do not pick one just because you have had a mail-shot through your door. Anyone who approaches you directly, in person or by phone, should be regarded with suspicion; reputable practitioners do not hawk for business.

Never be fooled by glossy brochures and impressive-looking credentials – they may mean nothing. Practitioners' diplomas and licences are not always genuine; even if they are, they may be of little or no value.

Many well-qualified practitioners advertise in *Yellow Pages,* in the same way that opticians, dentists and doctors do. But remember that anyone can be listed, so check the practitioner's qualifications with the organisation to which he or she claims to belong.

Membership of an organisation is, however, no guarantee of quality and good practice. You should check out the professional organisation. Find out how long it has been established. Some organisations are interested only in collecting the fee and have little or no idea of the quality and experience of the people on their books. Get a list of local practitioners from one of the 'umbrella' organisations (see Chapter 5).

Some organisations will send you a register of practitioners or give you names and addresses over the phone. Choosing a therapist who belongs to a reputable professional organisation is vital.

The best organisations will have the following safeguards:

- a set of educational and training standards
- a code of practice and ethics
- a complaints procedure

- disciplinary procedures, such as suspension or removal of the practitioner from the register
- a requirement for indemnity insurance, against malpractice or negligence claims.

Once you have found a practitioner, it is advisable to talk to him before you book an appointment. A good practitioner, far from objecting to your questions, will probably welcome them. If he refuses to answer them, look for another one. Ask yourself whether the practitioner seems warm, genuine and caring. Does he empathise with your condition? Does he seem sympathetic and trustworthy? Will you be able to confide in him? Does he seem hopeful about treating you?

Picking the right therapist ultimately depends on personal choice. You may, for example, prefer a practitioner of the same gender as yourself for therapies such as massage and osteopathy, where close physical contact is necessary. If you have a chronic condition, it may be that you will see the therapist once a month or once every two months for many years, so it is as important to have a good relationship with that person as it is with a solicitor or accountant. If you form a positive relationship with the therapist your chances of recovery should improve.

Questions to ask the practitioner:
- What are your methods of treatment? Are they appropriate to my condition?
- How many sessions might I need before I see any improvement?
- What are your qualifications and how long did you train for?
- How long have you been practising?
- To which professional body do you belong?
- Are you covered by professional indemnity insurance?
- How much will the treatment cost?

A good practitioner...
- welcomes your questions and answers them fully
- gives a full explanation of all the procedures involved in the treatment and tells you how you may feel afterwards

- tells you how much treatment will cost and gives you a rough estimate of how many treatment sessions you may need to have
- has had adequate training, will not have trained through a correspondence course and belongs to a recognised organisation
- does not guarantee recovery and tells you if he cannot help you
- has full professional indemnity insurance
- does not over-charge.

A bad practitioner...
- is rude, arrogant or offended when you ask questions
- promises to cure your condition (responsible practitioners, on the other hand, know that a cure cannot be guaranteed and that no medicine or therapy is 100 per cent effective)
- promises cures for specific conditions (responsible practitioners will say no more than that the treatment they are administering is sometimes successful in cases such as yours)
- tells you to stop seeing your doctor and/or to stop taking your medication
- does not listen to you or take a full case history – or, conversely, takes a prying, salacious interest in your personal life
- does not take notes
- rubbishes the work of other therapists and doctors
- makes you feel uneasy or uncomfortable
- tells you a lot of mumbo-jumbo. (Quacks might tell you, for example, that the body is a 'manifestation of a harmonic chord', that 'healing breakthroughs come through stepping into magic' and that you should 'unblock your channels and open yourself to healing and delight'. Compare this with 'osteopaths work with their hands using a range of treatment techniques' or 'the Alexander technique addresses the fundamental causes of many cases of back pain, neck and shoulder tension' and you will see the difference)
- charges far more (or far less) than other practitioners.

If, despite following these tips, you end up with a practitioner you are unhappy with and wish to complain about, you will find advice in Chapter 5 on how to do so.

At some stage in your treatment you must decide whether you wish to continue or not: a complementary therapist who receives fees from you for each session may not be as eager as, say, your NHS doctor to 'sign you off' once he or she feels the treatment has achieved its objective, and some may encourage you to continue with the therapy for far longer than necessary.

Opting for complementary medicine means being prepared to make your own decisions.

CHAPTER 2

COMPLEMENTARY MEDICINE AND THE NHS

COMPLEMENTARY medicine within the National Health Service has been marginalised despite the fact that the 1858 Medical Act did not prohibit non-orthodox or non-registered practitioners from treating patients provided they did not claim to be registered doctors, nor did the 1948 Act, which set up the NHS, explicitly preclude the practice of non-orthodox medicine within the NHS. For instance, homeopathy has been available under the NHS at five hospitals since 1948, but other complementary therapies have become available under the NHS only since the late 1980s.

The precise sum of money spent by the NHS on complementary medicine is not known. The Royal London Homoeopathic Hospital, which offers a range of complementary therapies under the NHS, received £2.6 million from health authorities and GP fundholders in 1995 alone. In 1996 the National Association of Health Authorities and Trusts (NAHAT) undertook a detailed study which aims to establish a national picture of the provision of complementary medicine within the NHS; the results will be published in late 1997.

Mainstream medical attitudes toward complementary medicine have been changing since the mid-1980s. In 1986 the British Medical Association (BMA) published a highly critical report, *Alternative therapy*, in which many therapies were dismissed as being untested, ineffective and potentially harmful. They were, it concluded, based on 'primitive beliefs and outmoded practices, almost all without basis', and their popularity was attributed to both the irrationality of consumers and the failure of doctors to address the wider needs of their patients.

Seven years later, however, the BMA produced *Complementary medicine: new approaches to good practice*. In it complementary medicine was referred to as 'non-conventional therapies', and the tone of the report was noticeably more balanced and conciliatory. The BMA had accepted that complementary medicine was more than just a passing phase, and decided to work with it.

Complementary medicine and GPs

In December 1991 Stephen Dorrell, then Parliamentary Secretary for Health, gave the green light for GPs to employ complementary therapists in their surgeries, provided the GPs retained clinical responsibility, or to use complementary medicine for treating patients themselves.

The popularity of complementary medicine is increasing in both hospitals (particularly among nurses), and GP practices (especially among fundholders). Many doctors are curious about complementary medicine; some practise it themselves. According to a study carried out by the University of Sheffield for the Department of Health in 1995, four in ten GPs in England provide access to some form of complementary therapy for their NHS patients. The study found that in one week 45 per cent of GPs recommended or endorsed the use of complementary therapies in their consultations, 21 per cent referred patients to a complementary therapist, both privately and under the NHS, and one in ten GPs treated patients with a complementary therapy themselves. However, although it would appear that many GPs are now offering complementary medicine, either themselves or through referral, the number of patients being offered these therapies is low; a study of GPs in Devon and Cornwall in 1995 revealed that although two-thirds of those interviewed were offering complementary therapies, on average only one patient per doctor per week was recommended to use them.

Modules in complementary therapy are now being incorporated into medical degrees, and are highly popular. In addition, the number of health-care professionals – doctors, nurses, physiotherapists, midwives and dentists – attending courses on how to integrate complementary therapies into their own practice has grown, and these people are taking their new skills back to their hospitals and clinics.

Complementary therapies in hospitals

Although not many hospitals offer complementary medicine, many nurses routinely incorporate it into their nursing practices; massage, aromatherapy and reflexology in particular are being used increasingly. Nurses are pioneering the expansion of complementary therapy in the NHS. The Royal College of Nursing has a Complementary Therapies Nursing Forum, with over 2,000 members, and nurses have spearheaded some 80 per cent of cases where policies for the practice of complementary therapies are being or have been developed in health services around Britain.

Some health authorities exclude complementary medicine on a policy basis while others are adopting a cautious approach. Very little is known about its use in hospitals in general because few of them, as yet, monitor the therapies they offer. Lewisham Hospital in south London is one of the few which does; its programme may indicate which complementary therapies will become more widely available in most hospitals in the future.

Local GPs refer almost 1,000 patients a year to the complementary therapy centre in Lewisham Hospital, and 26 GPs in the Lewisham, Lambeth and Southwark area have complementary therapy practitioners working with them in their surgeries. The centre offers outpatient treatment in osteopathy, acupuncture and homeopathy. It attracts 300-350 new referrals a year, many of them people suffering from back and musculo-skeletal problems, skin problems, upper respiratory problems, headaches and migraines. Their progress is being monitored carefully; the initial results suggest that those treated have improved while those on the waiting list have not.

All complementary practitioners at the hospital have to be registered with a recognised professional body and have at least three years' post-registration experience. The cost of the unit is £50,000 per year – about the same as that for three coronary heart bypass operations – which covers six appointments per patient, all remedies, the cost of a nurse to run the unit and payment for the practitioners. The hospital also has an outreach clinic based at a GP's surgery, with an acupuncturist visiting once a week. It also plans to set up a massage service for patients with life-threatening illnesses.

The Royal London Homoeopathic Hospital offers cancer patients homeopathic medicine to counteract the effects of radiotherapy, as well as Iskador therapy (treatment with mistletoe extract) and acupuncture, which are used alongside radiotherapy and chemotherapy. It also offers relaxation sessions, breathing awareness groups and pain management instruction, while nurses offer massage, shiatsu, reflexology and aromatherapy.

The hospital did a pilot study, published in 1995, of 50 breast cancer patients attending for the first time. It followed them for six months and found a significant reduction in both psychological distress and anxiety levels in the 21 patients who survived. It also found that women who were having drug therapy for breast cancer often had hot flushes, for which homeopathy, acupuncture and shiatsu provided relief.

Complementary medicine and care of elderly people

Health authorities are beginning to fund the use of complementary therapies in sheltered accommodation and residential homes for the elderly. The Central and Cecil Housing Trust in Richmond, Surrey, piloted a six-month study in 1994 into the use of complementary therapies with elderly people, funded by Age Concern and the local health authority (see also Aromatherapy). The project was independently monitored by a psychologist and lecturer in gerontology at Birkbeck College, University of London.

The residents were offered reflexology, aromatherapy, Japanese *reiki*, which involves the laying-on of hands, and relaxation. The therapies relieved many of the symptoms associated with old age – arthritis, sleeplessness, depression and dementia. Some residents had a good night's sleep for the first time in years and many seemed more cheerful and optimistic. The results were so dramatic that the trust has been inundated with requests for details from hundreds of residential homes.

At the time of writing the NHS is providing an increasing number of complementary therapies in response to patient demand.

However, as funding becomes increasingly scarce the NHS is being forced to prioritise the services it offers; those therapies which have scientific evidence to support them will be provided in preference to those which have not. Much work is going on to investigate the efficacy of complementary medicines, but until this has been done most of them will be available only privately.

CHAPTER 3

THE SCIENTIFIC CASE FOR COMPLEMENTARY MEDICINE

IT IS a common view that conventional medical trials cannot be conducted on unconventional therapies. Science and complementary medicine seem to be about very different things. Science is said to be about cold fact, the accurate measurement of the material world; it reduces everything to its constituent parts. Complementary medicine is said to be about recognising the spiritual and emotional aspects of health, factors which are difficult to take apart or measure. In addition, the language of, say, an acupuncturist, and that of an anatomist appear to be completely different: nowhere in an orthodox medical textbook will one find acupuncture points or 'meridians'.

The usual method for doctors and scientists to investigate the value of a treatment is to conduct a 'randomised controlled trial' (RCT), whereby a group of patients is assigned at random to receive one of two different treatments. Doctors then measure whether the patients improve and compare the results in the different groups. A 'double-blind' RCT is a test in which patients receive either a real drug or a placebo (see Glossary) and neither they nor the researchers know which is which.

There has been much debate about whether the RCT could be applied to complementary therapies. Some people argue that RCTs cannot be used because it is difficult to design suitable placebos: you can certainly give a patient a fake drug, but how do you give him a fake massage or acupuncture treatment? Others maintain that the RCT requires every patient to receive identical treatment, whereas in many complementary therapies different approaches are used for different patients. Another argument is that what is important is how patients feel, and what their quality of life is, not what can be measured with scales, rulers and test tubes.

However, many of these arguments depend on a misunderstanding of the RCT. An RCT does not need a placebo group. In fact, placebos are not possible for the majority of conventional therapies: most of what surgeons, nurses or physiotherapists do could not be tested in a placebo-controlled trial. Moreover, patients in an RCT do not have to receive identical treatments. For example, surgeons always vary what they do depending on the individual patient, yet RCTs can and have been conducted on surgery. In addition, it is not necessary to use laboratory measurements in an RCT. In most trials, questionnaires designed to measure pain, anxiety or quality of life are used to determine how the patient feels.

So the usual methods of investigating therapies can be adapted to complementary medicine. Perhaps the best proof of this is that many RCTs have been conducted in therapies as diverse as acupuncture, spiritual healing, yoga, fasting and reflexology.

The main problem with research into complementary medicine has not been theoretical issues of experimental design – although many studies in the area suffer from the weakness of having very few subjects – but practical issues such as funding and research skills. Very little money has been spent on complementary medicine research. Much of the funding is available only for research on drugs and other conventional therapies. That said, throwing money at the problem will not necessarily solve it. Few complementary practitioners have the knowledge or experience to conduct high-quality research, so it is doubtful whether a large amount of research funding could be spent wisely. What seems to be needed is a long-term investment in research, not just for trials but for developing skills and institutional resources. Such investment would benefit everyone who needs to make decisions on complementary medicine, including patients.

Does it work?

Perhaps the most common question asked about complementary medicine is 'Does it work?'. However, this may not be the most appropriate question.

First, what does the 'it' refer to? Is it complementary medicine as a whole or a particular therapy? Is it the specific technique, such as inserting needles or giving herbal pills, or the treatment as a whole, including the practitioner's time, care and attention? The meaning of the verb 'work' is also open to interpretation. If a therapy is said to 'work' only if it cures a disease, then this seems to ignore important issues such as relief from pain or quality of life. On the other hand, a therapy might be said to work if the patient feels better. What view would be taken if someone with cancer enjoyed an improved mood and sense of well-being after treatment but died shortly afterwards?

Critics of complementary medicine often claim that the effectiveness of therapies which have little or no scientific evidence behind them is due to the placebo effect, whereby people feel better simply *because* they are taking medication or some other form of treatment for their condition. This is dismissive not just of complementary medicine, but also of the placebo effect, the power of which orthodox medicine is only just beginning to recognise and harness.

Research generally aims to answer questions which are very much more specific than 'Does it work?' and it is often difficult to come to general conclusions on the basis of individual studies. That said, a brief overview of the research literature can provide at least some help in assessing the value of complementary therapies.

Acupuncture

A multitude of studies has been conducted on acupuncture. The evidence suggests that acupuncture is probably not just a placebo: in one set of trials,[1] stimulation of an acupuncture point on the wrist was found to be very much more effective for nausea than stimulating false acupuncture points. Studies showing that acupuncture can affect animals, even those under anaesthetic,[2] provide further evidence that the reason acupuncture works is not just because people believe in it. Some of the basic principles of acupuncture have been proved to be valid. For example, researchers found that the electrical resistance of acupuncture points corresponding to the heart is different in patients suffering from heart problems from what it is in healthy people.[3] As is the case with many complementary therapies, less research has been undertaken on the long-term effects of acupuncture and whether it is better than other forms of treatment.

Homeopathy

Many homeopathic remedies are so dilute that they do not contain even a single molecule of active ingredient. Most research has been directed at determining whether homeopathy is different in any way from a placebo. In the early 1990s, a group of Dutch researchers obtained and analysed all studies on homeopathy that they could identify. Their findings, which were published in the *British Medical Journal,*[4] were favourable: 81 out of 105 trials were positive. The majority of even the most rigorous, double-blind studies found homeopathy to be superior to a placebo. The reviewers concluded that 'the evidence of clinical trials is positive but not sufficient to draw definitive conclusions'.

Osteopathy and chiropractic

Osteopathy and chiropractic are similar enough to be considered together for the purposes of research. There is considerable evidence that manipulation of the spine is of benefit for back and neck pain.[5-8] However, it is not known whether any one form of manipulation – osteopathy, chiropractic or physiotherapy – is more effective than any other. Furthermore, there is evidence against some of the other claims made by practitioners: for example, that treatment is of benefit for asthma[9] or hypertension.[10]

Herbal medicine

Many pharmaceutical drugs are based on herbal products, so it is not surprising that some herbs have been found to be of benefit for specific conditions. There is evidence, for example, that ginger can treat morning sickness[11] and that an extract from St John's wort (hypericum) is an effective treatment for depression.[12] However, herbalists do not usually prescribe single herbs for single diseases. Very little evidence exists to show whether what herbalists do in practice is of benefit.

Hypnotherapy

Evidence has shown that hypnotherapy is of benefit for asthma,[13] irritable bowel syndrome[14] and some types of headache.[15] However, it is curious that hypnotherapy does not seem to be a good treatment for patients who want to stop smoking.[16] The biggest difficulty in interpreting such studies is that hypnotherapy covers many techniques and an individual practitioner may not use the same techniques as those used in the trial. In such instances, it is impossible to be sure that the treatment will produce the same results.

Nutritional approaches

Some complementary practitioners prescribe high-dose vitamins and unusual diets. At the time of writing no evidence exists on the benefits of these nutritional approaches as a whole. It is known that some diets are not effective. In one study, a special arthritis regime known as the 'Dong diet' was found to be no better than a diet chosen at random.[17] However, one particular approach, known as elimination dieting or the food intolerance diet, has been shown to be effective in the treatment of a variety of conditions including rheumatoid arthritis,[18] migraine[19] and hyperactivity in children.[20]

Massage and aromatherapy

Few people doubt that massage is a relaxing experience and there is strong evidence that it can reduce anxiety. In one trial, a group of adolescents in a psychiatric unit were given massage. They demonstrated much greater reduction in anxiety than those who watched videotapes.[21] Gentle foot massage has also been shown to be of benefit for patients in intensive care.[22] However, practitioners make many other claims about massage – for example, that it can relieve pain or reduce blood pressure – yet there is little evidence on whether it really has these effects. Research on aromatherapy is even more limited. Some studies suggest that certain oils can alleviate conditions such as acne[23] or athlete's foot[24] but there is little evidence that the use of essential oils for massage provides any benefit greater than a pleasant smell.

Other therapies

There is also reliable evidence that some complementary practices are *not* of value. Studies have been undertaken on allergy clinics, which typically claim to diagnose allergies or nutritional deficiencies by analysing samples of hair.[25,26] Such clinics often reported different results for hair from the same individual. Moreover, though they diagnosed all sorts of allergies and deficiencies in healthy individuals, they failed to identify them in people with known allergies. Both iridology[27,28] and kinesiology[29] have been shown to be ineffective.

Summary

Though it might seem at first that it would be difficult to conduct scientific trials on complementary therapies, this can and has been done. A body of evidence has been amassed to show that each of the main therapies can be effective for at least some conditions. Some techniques have been proved to be ineffective and should be avoided. That said, it cannot be doubted that there has been insufficient research on complementary therapies. Many important questions remain unanswered, including those concerning the long-term effect of treatment and the issue of which therapy might be most appropriate in a given condition. Greater investment in complementary medicine research is needed in order to inform consumer choice.

CHAPTER 4

COMPLEMENTARY MEDICINE: THE GOOD, THE BAD AND THE UNKNOWN

COMPLEMENTARY medicine is an area in which there are still many unanswered questions. Little of it has been tested satisfactorily, and most of the evidence to support it is anecdotal. Not surprisingly, therefore, many myths still surround it. This chapter examines some of the good and bad points about complementary medicine, looks at basic concepts common to some therapies and dispels the most common misconceptions.

Advantages of complementary medicine

The reasons why people turn to complementary medicine, which were looked at in Chapter 1, are both negative (such as disillusionment with aspects of conventional medicine) and positive (the fact that so many people claim to have benefited from it). The perceived advantages include the holistic approach taken by most therapists, who recognise that the mind and body influence each other strongly; and the control over their health and treatment which complementary therapies give to their users.

Holism

Therapists who practise holism examine each patient as a complete person: lifestyle, relationships, diet and occupation, for example, are all taken into consideration. The holistic approach is essential to the treatment. Many therapists believe that the state of the mind and spirit is just as important as the condition of the body.

Although doctors would also like to think that they look at their patients as whole people, time restrictions usually prevent them from doing so. GPs usually spend a couple of minutes talking to each patient before writing out a prescription. In mainstream medicine patients can sometimes feel dehumanised – treated as biological entities, such as a badly behaved uterus or a poorly functioning heart or another piece of corporeal plumbing that is not working properly. It is for this reason, as well as lack of communication between patient and GP, that many people look for alternatives to orthodox treatments.

Most initial sessions with a complementary practitioner will take an hour, during which time the patient will be asked questions about all areas of his or her life. Because therapists spend this time talking to their patients, they generally have good interpersonal skills. They also tend to talk to patients using language that they understand rather than in medical jargon. However, the ability to listen to and empathise with patients is now being taught in medical school, and doctors' skills at dealing with patients' emotions and idiosyncrasies are improving.

Complementary therapists know the importance of touch; its healing power has been demonstrated by several studies which show that patients who have had physical contact with their nurses get better more quickly than patients who have not; in a 1988 paper, a Macmillan Cancer Fund lecturer concluded that touch is an essential part of patient care. According to the author, the evidence indicates that direct contact can facilitate communication and promote comfort and well-being.

The holistic approach is beneficial because patients feel more positive if they know someone is taking an interest in them as people, not just as biomedical problems, and is really listening to them. Critics of the holistic approach may regard it as self-indulgent flattery, or 'tea and sympathy', but for the chronically ill it is often very effective. Doctors who are aware of this may consider recommending their 'difficult' patients to complementary therapists.

The mind-body link

The mind-body link is so important to complementary therapists that they regard it as essential to take the time to explore which psychological factors, if any, have been instrumental in causing an illness. Mainstream practitioners have also recognised for some time that psychological factors influence disease, but they are only now beginning to realise the impact that the mind and emotions can have on the body, and *vice versa*. In recognition of this, a new research field – psychoneuroimmunology – has been flourishing in the United States since the mid-1980s and became established in the UK in the early 1990s.

There is increasing evidence that the personality of an individual can modify the immune response: for example, people of a cheery, positive disposition may be less likely to be ill than people who are more negative.

The immune system is a complex defence mechanism against viruses and bacteria. Research has shown that stress, particularly severe stress, such as that triggered by bereavement or the breakdown of a marriage, has marked biochemical and hormonal effects within the body. Nevertheless, no research suggests that stress or being depressed cause cancer of themselves.

Scientists have shown that complementary therapies which involve relaxation, meditation, hypnotherapy and other psychological interventions may be able to boost the immune system in cancer patients and prolong survival. In addition, several studies have suggested that social support has a significant impact on the survival rate of cancer patients. In a study published in *The Lancet* in October 1989, researchers monitored a group of women with breast cancer. Half met on an informal basis to chat and offer each other support; those in the other group did not. The women who got together and supported each other survived twice as long.

Patient involvement

The medical profession often finds chronic illnesses difficult to deal with because the causes, and therefore the treatments, are not always obvious; doctors either issue repeat prescriptions for drugs which may not be effective and which may have unpleasant side-effects, or simply tell the patient there is nothing they can do. It is at this stage that many patients feel that they want to do something positive to help themselves instead of stoically accepting the affliction: turning to complementary therapies is a way of achieving this. Complementary medicine can offer a way of living more comfortably with a disorder even if it cannot provide a cure for it.

Drawbacks of the complementary approach

Complementary medicine, like any system of treatment, has disadvantages too. The view taken by many therapists that we are all capable of achieving and maintaining good health, and that we are in a sense responsible for any illness we have, is problematic. This and other unsatisfactory aspects of complementary medicine are discussed below.

Total health

Many complementary practitioners maintain that everyone has the potential to achieve total health. They believe that all illnesses are caused by an unhealthy lifestyle, environment and negative emotions, all of which are theoretically within our control to change. Some even think that cancer takes hold as a direct result of repressed anger or a bout of depression; there is no evidence for this, although research shows that some cancer patients who receive support from friends and family tend to recover faster or at least live longer than those who do not.

The goal of total health is in fact misplaced. Some people will never be able to attain it, because of their constitution or their genes. In addition, most people develop illness because, by chance, they catch viruses or are invaded by bacteria. Although we are all more susceptible to illness when we are in low spirits, no evidence has shown that being depressed or in an emotional turmoil affects the immune system to the extent that an individual can become seriously ill.

Complementary therapists believe that by living in as healthy a way as possible, i.e. by taking exercise, eating sensibly, not smoking or drinking, and by getting to grips with negative emotions, everyone can achieve harmony and total health. In some cases this is true; staying fit and eating healthily may well help people ward off colds and 'flu, as well as illnesses caused by the excesses of modern living. However, the same cannot be said for diabetes or epilepsy, for example, which may be present from birth.

Other criticisms of the complementary approach

A corollary of the belief that it is in the power of everybody to achieve total health is that a person who is not well is in some way responsible for his or her illness. Some therapists maintain that mental attitudes affect the progress of a disease: if someone is not getting well, it could be because he or she does not have the right attitude to the illness. This in turn could make the individual feel guilty, which can hardly be helpful (see Fighting cancer, below).

Another problem with this approach is that it locates the illness and treatment within the individual rather than society: complementary therapists do not address the issues of inequality and poverty, and the consequent lack of satisfactory housing, inadequate hygiene and poor diet, which are the biggest causes of disease. Conventional medicine at least tries to educate people about the importance of a healthy diet and good hygiene.

Although reputable therapists would advise patients to carry on with conventional treatment for their conditions, a few are antagonistic towards modern medicine and science. Occasionally, people using complementary medicine may themselves share that opinion, and either not visit a GP at all or discontinue medical treatment. Complementary medicine can be extremely harmful if it is used as a substitute for proper diagnosis and treatment. Doctors spend years learning not just about anatomy and physiology but how to diagnose disorders. People may be put at risk by practitioners who are not adequately trained to recognise and manage a disease for which there is a good mainstream treatment. A case was reported in 1994 in which four insulin-dependent diabetics either reduced or stopped their intake of insulin in favour of therapeutic approaches, including prayer, faith healing, unusual diets and supplements of vitamins and trace elements. Three of them contracted ketoacidosis, a potentially serious condition in which excessive amounts of ketones accumulate in the body. (Ketones are chemical substances produced from the imperfect oxidation of fats and protein foods, which may be caused by eating too little or by inadequately controlled diabetes.) In one case it became life-threatening. The fourth person suffered weight loss and hyperglycaemia (abnormally high level of glucose in the blood). One of the patients developed a serious disease of the retina.

Health, illness and theories of the body

Practitioners of some systems of complementary medicine view the body differently from the way in which conventional (Western) medicine does. Terms such as 'blocked energy', 'meridians' and 'toxins' may seem incomprehensible, but are essential to the understanding of how their therapies are meant to work.

Blocked and unblocked energy

The concept of energy is fundamental to many complementary therapies. In science, there are several different definitions of energy; complementary practitioners sometimes use yet another, completely different, idea of energy. They maintain that energy or a vital force flows around the body: when it is blocked or imbalanced it can lead to ill-health. Some therapies are based on complex concepts of how the energy circulates. It is not yet known whether this sort of energy really exists or whether it is just a metaphor for what is supposed to happen during treatment. In traditional Chinese medicine this 'vital force' is called qi (pronounced 'chee'). It is said to flow along invisible pathways called meridians, of which there are 12 main ones. In yoga the 'life force' is called prana and the pathways along which it is said to flow are called nadis. When the energy becomes blocked, deficient or 'stagnant', illness is said to result.

Acupuncture aims to unblock the meridians by placing needles on specific points along them. Yoga is said to invigorate the seven chakras, which are said to be points of focused energy, and to unblock the prana. Most complementary therapies aim to unblock energy in some way, thereby healing the patient. However, when energy is said to flow round the body or from a healer to a patient, no changes of any kind occur that can be measured; for this reason some doctors remain sceptical.

Body energy

Physical energy, on the other hand, can be measured. Bodies emit electromagnetic energy, measurable by taking an electrocardio-graph (ECG) of the heart, an electromyogram (EMG) which gauges the condition of the muscles, and an electroencephalogram (EEG) of the brain waves. The body also gives off thermal or heat energy, as well as sound and light. This electromagnetic energy can now be measured up to a distance of 50cm around the body by means of a sophisticated piece of computer equipment called a magnetometer.

A remarkable finding is that the energy given off by the heart is 40-50 times greater than that emitted by the brain, making it the dominant energy source in the body. The energy emitted by the heart flows through every cell in the body, and researchers have now discovered that energy radiating from the heart varies dramat-ically depending on what sort of mood the patient is in. Scientists have shown that there can be an energy transfer from one person to another. During experiments to measure the brainwave of one person and the heartbeat of another, they found that when the lat-ter person touched the former, the heartbeat was picked up on the brainwave monitor.

Some researchers believe that the healthy body is one that is perfectly 'entrained' – in other words, all the energy sources are working in harmony. Animals have a habit of being influenced by each other in strange ways. It is a well-known phenomenon that women living together menstruate at the same time, shoals of fish turn at the same time, and flocks of birds move as one; after a while even clock pendulums will swing together.

It is possible to become 'entrained' by another person. If some-one is in a positive state of mind, another person can become entrained with positive feelings. Corporate teams can be entrained to work in a positive way, and some complementary practitioners believe they can entrain their clients to their own healthier, more powerful bodies.

Although one person's energy field can be picked up by another and we can control the sort of energy we emit by meditation, visualisation or stress-relieving tactics, it has not been scientifically proved that one person's energy can *alter* the energy of another. So how can it happen? An explanation may come from the concept of subtle energy.

Subtle energy

Practitioners of complementary medicine claim that energy also works at a subtle level, i.e. it is there and works but it is immeasurable. Quantum and particle physicists maintain that matter and energy, given the right conditions, can interchange. The atomic bomb shows that when you blow up matter it turns into vast amounts of energy. A molecule, comprising a nucleus and its electrons, is merely a minute amount of energy whirling around.

Complementary therapists would argue that matter is not matter as such but energy. Therefore, according to them, our bodies can be viewed as being energy systems, which can get out of balance, resulting in disease. They believe they can influence the body at a basic energy level and get it to right itself. However, this is impossible to prove. Anecdotal evidence exists to suggest that therapies that claim to heal through manipulation of this subtle energy may be successful. Complementary practitioners believe that the body, given the right conditions, will always heal itself. However, although many conditions do get better by themselves, the idea that the body 'heals itself' is dangerously simplistic. Diabetes, for example, is caused by a deficiency of insulin and no amount of unblocking of energy channels will rectify the situation. In this case, if the body were left to sort itself out, the person would die.

Toxins

Some complementary therapists, particularly colonic hydrotherapists (who practise what is popularly known as colonic irrigation), naturopaths, iridologists, some massage therapists and aromatherapists, maintain that the human body is full of toxins imbibed from the food we eat and the polluted atmosphere in which we live and work; they disapprove of coffee, tea, sugar and processed foods, as well as nicotine and alcohol. Iridologists try to dissuade people from eating foods which contain or create toxins: these include meat (including poultry), fish, refined white flour products, refined sugars, artificial additives, colourings, preservatives and hard cheeses. The sole aim of certain therapies is to rid people of toxins; colons, we are told, need to be flushed out and only organic food should be eaten. Constipation is seen as the epitome of toxicity.

The notion that the body is a repository for toxins was particularly popular in the late nineteenth and early twentieth centuries. Sir William Arbuthnot Lane, an eminent consulting surgeon at Guy's Hospital, London, described the colon as 'a veritable Pandora's box out of which comes more human misery, suffering, mental and moral as well as physical, than from any other known source'. This theory fell out of favour in mainstream medicine after the Second World War but is still popular with some complementary therapists.

It is true that too much coffee, alcohol and fatty foods are not good for the body and most people would benefit from cutting down on them. It would also be foolish to deny that what we eat has an impact on our health. Heart disease, bowel disorders and tooth decay are linked to the foods we eat. However, a diet that consists of a balance of vegetables, fruit, moderate amounts of protein, carbohydrates and fat is perfectly healthy and will not cause any problems. A daily glass of wine has also been found to protect people from heart disease.

The kidneys, colon and liver deal very effectively with any toxins that do enter the body, which, in any case, come from organic vegetables as well as meat and processed foods.

Fasting can help some conditions. Research has shown that fasting and a vegetarian diet have proved effective in the treatment of rheumatoid arthritis. However, not eating properly can also cause blood-sugar levels to fall, resulting in headaches; this is not a sign of toxins being eliminated from the body, as some therapists would suggest, but an indication that the body needs sugar.

In addition, the body relies on its accumulation of carbohydrate and fat if it is not getting enough food. The metabolism has to adjust in order to use them. Body fat is a store for fat-soluble chemicals, so when the body starts losing weight these chemicals will enter the bloodstream, increasing the level of toxins.

Toxins are not, as some therapists would like their clients to believe, a problem: and it can even be dangerous to follow a strict diet which has been designed to 'cleanse' the body; eat sensibly, and the body should stay healthy.

Misconceptions

Complementary medicine appeals to people for various reasons, not all of which are valid. Believing that a therapy is good for one merely because it is either 'natural' or 'old' is unwise.

'Natural' equals 'safe'

Complementary medicine is popular partly because it is seen as natural and non-invasive. Its remedies are made from naturally occurring plants and oils which are generally regarded as safe compared with the synthetic, laboratory-produced chemicals used in mainstream treatments; also, they have few unpleasant side-effects. Products for complementary medicine are often packaged in green, perhaps bearing a delicate illustration of a flower or other plant, or a photograph of surf: images of nature that are familiar and non-threatening.

However, natural substances are not always safe; deadly night-shade, rhubarb leaves and uncooked kidney beans can kill, as can many berries and mushrooms. Some herbal tonics have been found to be poisonous or contaminated (such products do not have to undergo the same rigorous tests as mainstream medicines, which have to be licensed by the Medicines Control Agency; see Chinese herbal medicine and Herbal medicine). Nevertheless, the number of people who have died as a direct result of taking complementary medicine is low compared with deaths related to the taking of conventional medicine.

To say that only 'natural' treatments are beneficial would be wrong and dangerous. Scientists have spent years developing many successful life-saving drugs and techniques. In many cases synthetic drugs are far more effective than complementary treatments. In fact, a world without man-made medicines would mean life with numerous diseases, more women would die in childbirth, and disorders such as epilepsy and diabetes would not be controlled; life expectancy would be much shorter. So the epithet of 'natural', in isolation, is in fact far from being a guarantee of goodness, or of effectiveness. Complementary medicine should be used alongside mainstream medicine, not as a substitute for it (see Other criticisms, above).

'Ancient' equals 'good'

The fact that many complementary therapies have their roots in ancient practices – from Egypt, India, China and Japan, for example – and have therefore stood the test of time, also attracts people to them. 'Old', like 'natural', is often thought to mean 'good'. Although some ancient treatments do have some merit (for example, t'ai chi is calming and acupuncture relieves pain), others, such as blood-letting, are completely ineffective and have been abandoned. There is no reason why an ancient therapy should be more effective or better for you than a modern one.

The patient's experience

Many people who receive complementary therapy are happy with their treatment; however, some derive little benefit and others are unhappy about their experience.

Usually their disappointment comes not from the fact that the therapy they tried did not work, but because it raised their hopes and expectations and robbed them of precious time and money. The following stories illustrate the sorts of success and failure that may result.

Case study 1: fighting cancer

Alexander Moore from Northern Ireland was diagnosed in 1990 with testicular cancer; the tumour, testicle and some of his lymph glands were removed but a year later doctors found that the cancer had returned; this time it had spread into the abdominal organs, into the bowel and through the bones and muscles. He was treated with chemotherapy and radiotherapy, which prolonged his life for another year. However, he then got secondary cancer in his spine, shoulder, ribs and liver. In March 1993 he died, aged 32.

Throughout his illness, Alexander had put his trust in complementary practitioners.

'Alexander had been a believer in homeopathy before he became ill, so he was having homeopathy, plus all the conventional stuff,' recalls his widow, Pat. 'But then he began seeing more therapists, always recommended by the therapist he had last seen. He was young and vital and lived every moment to the full. To be told your quality of life is seriously threatened and that the length of it is quite probably shortened was terrible. He was trying to fight against his illness as best he could.'

Mr Moore tried cranial osteopathy, massage, aromatherapy, Bach flower remedies and a strong herbal tonic called Hoxsey medicine. He even went to see a psychic surgeon, who said that a demon would 'dematerialise' the tumour.

'Alexander tried a number of nutritional therapies – drinking lots of broccoli juice and taking vitamin supplements. Then he tried exclusion diets, cutting out pork, tomatoes, tea, coffee, alcohol and anything with preservatives in it. That left grilled white meat, mainly chicken, and fish and organic vegetables, preferably raw.

'And all this was urged on someone who had a major abdominal tumour whose system wasn't working well. The conventional doctors said he could eat anything he wanted. They said he needed all the nutrition he could get. These people were starving him.'

The Moores also visited 'healers' who said they could pass their hands over the body and 'feel' the sickness and work on it. The healers charged £20 an hour. Altogether, the Moores spent several thousand pounds.

'The only effect I felt these therapists had was one of false hope,' continues Mrs Moore. 'None of them said, "We're sorry you're terminally ill and we'll help you come to terms with it." What they said was "There's no such thing as terminal, your life is up to you, you can communicate with your cancer and reverse it. It can even go away." They said he was to blame for his own illness.

'He used to come back from these sessions thinking he was going to beat it and refusing to take his morphine. When you are high, after a faith-healing session or a football match or in a spiritual church, you get wildly excited, have a rush of hormones and you don't feel pain for a while. But it doesn't last and when it doesn't work out you feel betrayed.

'Some therapies, like massage, were wonderful. When you've got a terrible illness like cancer, you feel awful. You want to take this terrible thing out of your body and throw it away and you can't. And for someone to touch you and show that they care about you is an amazing thing.'

Mrs Moore feels strongly that the fact that the vast majority of complementary therapies are unregulated means that scrupulous and unscrupulous practitioners can practise side by side.

'At the moment, you can't tell the good practitioners from the bad ones. They can tell you anything they want and not be responsible for the consequences, and the consequences for my husband were bad. We spent our time chasing mirages.'

Case study 2: coping with a back injury

Eugenie Warner started to visit a chiropractor, Christopher Turner, after she suffered injuries that did not heal for a while. She was a police officer and had been badly beaten up in 1988 while on duty, when she was dragged along the pavement by the neck and kicked in the back, as well as having five teeth kicked out. The teeth were replaced and she thought the nagging pain in her back was due to bruising and would eventually go away. But it persisted down the lower left side of her back.

'I was in the most appalling pain,' she recalls. 'My doctor sent me to see a physiotherapist, but it was like scratching the surface and nothing happened. I thought I would give chiropractic a try.'

Mr Turner examined her, talked to her at length and simply clicked her back into place. 'It was like a weight being lifted from my back. The relief was instantaneous – quite amazing. It did ache afterwards, but that was because my muscles had been in spasm and it took time to get back to normal. I had to go back twice a week for the first couple of weeks and now I go along every couple of months.'

Then Mrs Warner was knocked off her police motorcycle and injured her neck, and Mr Turner successfully treated that too. Chiropractic also eases her occasional migraine. 'They normally start with a build-up of stress around the neck and shoulders and if

I'm feeling particularly wound up I go along to Christopher or the aromatherapist who works at his clinic, and this relaxes me and eases the neck problems.

'Once I visited him with a terrible migraine. I was feeling sick, saw flashing lights and had all the typical symptoms. I had to be driven to the clinic, but when I left, all I had was a mild headache. My neck had been wound up and tight, and he just clicked it and the migraine lifted.'

Mrs Warner was referred by her GP and her treatment – £25 a session – was paid for by a private health insurance company. 'I think it's money well spent and my GP thinks the treatment is marvellous. He's just happy that one of his patients is being well looked after.'

CHAPTER 5

COMPLEMENTARY MEDICINE AND THE LAW

IN BRITAIN there is little direct regulation of non-medically qualified practitioners. Under common law all complementary therapists can practise freely and do more or less what they want, subject only to minor legislation. Anyone, regardless of qualifications or experience, can set up as a homeopath, reflexologist, aromatherapist or massage practitioner – for example, screw a brass plate to the front door and open shop. He can perfume his 'clinic' with essential oils, hang 'certificates', which may or may not be worth the paper they are printed on, on the wall, invent a string of letters to put after his name and play New Age whalesongs, while he pockets customers' hard-earned money. This is completely legal but, for people who are emotionally vulnerable, extremely dangerous.

The only legislation there is forbids non-medically qualified practitioners to claim to be a state-registered professional, such as a dentist, doctor or physiotherapist, or to be able to cure certain medical conditions, such as cancer, diabetes, epilepsy, tuberculosis and venereal disease.

Although complementary medicine is generally far safer than mainstream medicine, it does carry risks. Hundreds of cases of adverse effects from complementary therapies have been reported worldwide, including some deaths, and the highest risk comes from unqualified practitioners.

However, most complementary therapies have registering bodies, through which you can check that the person treating you is fully qualified in his field, though it is important to find out about the therapy first. Spending five years learning about a treatment which is essentially nonsense does not make the treatment any more worthy or efficacious, although it does mean that the practitioner will probably stick to a code of practice and ethics.

It can also be tempting to visit someone who has been recommended by a friend, but before you do, check the practitioner's credentials (see Chapter 1).

The number of complementary practitioners has been expanding in Britain by an estimated 10 per cent per year since the mid-1980s, in response to the large and ever-increasing public demand. This flood of potential patients seeking complementary therapy has encouraged some practitioners, such as osteopaths and chiropractors, to regulate their own therapies.

The Osteopaths Act 1993 and the Chiropractors Act 1994 have given these two therapies the benefits of state regulation. Other therapies, such as acupuncture and homeopathy, may well follow suit. The regulation of other therapies still needs to be improved. Each therapy should have a single registering body, and consumers should be able to trust a practitioner's registration as proof that they are reputable.

Increasingly, practitioners have grown to realise that if they are to continue enjoying the common-law freedom to practise that characterises complementary medicine in Britain they must get their house in order. Much more emphasis is now being placed on qualifications, training, and registration with an organisation which the public can see is *bona fide* and which has codes of practice and ethics.

In the meantime, because this transformation is happening very slowly, the consumer is faced with a bewildering number of registering bodies for each therapy. Many have impressive-sounding names, such as the International Association of X or the British Council for Y, but there are no guidelines as to which ones are genuine and which ones are 'better' than others.

Most of these bodies have elaborate codes of practice and ethics, and if a practitioner fails to abide by them he can be struck off, but this is not comparable to a doctor being struck off by the General Medical Council (GMC). Because medicine is regulated by the state, a doctor has to register with the GMC before he can practise. If subsequently a complaint is made against that doctor and he is found guilty of serious professional misconduct, the GMC's ultimate sanction would be to have that doctor struck off and his name erased from the register. It would then be a criminal offence for that doctor to practise within the NHS and write out NHS prescriptions (although he could still write out private prescriptions), and if such a doctor were found practising he would be prosecuted.

Being 'struck off' is not as serious for a complementary practitioner; having been ousted from a particular association one week, he could easily join another organisation the following week and open for business again legally.

Umbrella organisations representing complementary medicine

The growth of complementary therapies has prompted the formation of several umbrella organisations, founded between 1981 and 1990. These represent the interests of practitioners, which may not necessarily be those of consumers. Two main bodies have been established, as well as various campaigning groups.

The **British Complementary Medicine Association (BCMA)** was set up in 1990 and is the largest overall body. It claims to represent about 26,000 practitioners in 50 organisations covering 30 therapies. Its aim is to encourage the diverse organisations of individual therapies to join together into single therapy groups and act collectively.

The organisations, not individuals who belong to them, pay to be on the register it runs, and members of the public can contact the BCMA either to check on the qualifications of a practitioner or to find a qualified therapist in a particular field who practises in their area. Each therapy belongs to a 'therapy group' within the BCMA, which dictates what qualifications are needed for membership, and practitioners must fulfil the criteria laid down by the group.

The BCMA is a non-profit-making organisation. Its committee members are elected annually and are unpaid, so they claim that the BCMA is more independent than the Institute of Complementary Medicine, which is run by two paid directors.

The **Institute for Complementary Medicine (ICM)** was established as a charity in 1982 to provide information for the public about complementary practitioners. It represents nearly 800 organisations in the field and has about 2,000 therapists covering approximately 18 therapies on its British Register of Complementary Practitioners.

In addition, the **Council for Complementary and Alternative Medicine (CCAM)**★ provides a forum for communication and co-operation between professional bodies representing acupuncture, herbal medicine, homeopathy, naturopathy and osteopathy. It was set up to support the professional development of these five disciplines and to promote public knowledge of good-quality complementary care.

The **Natural Medicines Society (NMS)**★ was set up in 1985 to protect the consumers' right to have access to high-quality alternative treatment and it works to ensure that natural medicines are safe and produced to a high standard. Claiming that complementary medicine is still under threat, it has embarked on a campaign to safeguard such medicine from 'ill-informed interference' and to push for high standards of training. To this end, it has set up a Medicines Advisory Research Committee, which can be called upon by government bodies for advice.

Both the CCAM and the NMS lobby on behalf of complementary therapies when the latter are threatened by adverse legislation. Both have close links with the All-Party Parliamentary Group for Alternative and Complementary Medicine and have occasional meetings with ministers. This active parliamentary group is a forum for the exchange of views promoting 'sensible' policies on complementary medicine. Two major debates on the subject have taken place in the House of Lords, the first in May 1990 and the second in January 1996, when peers called on the government to support complementary medicine by funding research.

However, the government's attitude towards complementary medicine, described as 'benevolent neutrality', is unlikely to change. Although it supports the right of complementary practitioners to practise, it neither encourages nor discourages its use.

Regulation of complementary medicine

The government shows no enthusiasm for regulating the whole industry but it encourages specific professional groups, such as osteopathy and chiropractic, to regulate themselves; a health professional is defined under Section 2 of the Access to Health Records Act 1990 as a registered medical practitioner. Ministers are unlikely to change their stance.

The government is caught between two stools: the right of individuals to exercise their own choice in health care; and the need to protect consumers not only against bogus practitioners, but against harm.

At the time of writing, the government maintains that it is not necessary for the state to regulate the industry because there is no evidence that complementary therapies harm people. At the same time, it is unlikely to regulate something that has neither hard scientific evidence to back it up nor the full support of the medical establishment (despite a favourable report by the BMA, see Chapter 1), let alone the powerful drugs industry lobby.

In short, there is no compulsion for the government to regulate complementary therapies by statute. Instead, it encourages self-regulation.

In addition, unlike osteopathy and chiropractic, most of the complementary therapies are not ready for legislation. Herbalism, acupuncture and homeopathy are almost ready, i.e. they have enough scientific evidence to back up their claims, but most therapies are dominated by large numbers of rival organisations. However, without proper legislation and protection of title, the consumer will always be short-changed.

Complementary therapies and continental Europe

A report on complementary medicine drafted by the Belgian Green MEP Paul Lannoye was presented to the European Union Committee on the Environment, Public Health and Consumer Protection in April 1996. The report calls for freedom for consumers in Europe to choose what type of treatment they want, while appropriate guarantees for their safety are ensured. These guarantees could be obtained through higher standards of training for practitioners, which should be harmonised throughout the EU, and through high-quality manufacturing procedures for all health-care products. This would mean the establishment of recognised professional bodies for each individual complementary therapy in each member state, similar to the British General Osteopathic Council (GOsC), although, unlike the GOsC, the bodies concerned would not have to be enshrined in statute. Such a structure would allow for mutual recognition between member states and the movement of therapists around Europe.

Britain is unique in that consumers have access to systems of medicine that most other European citizens do not have, such as herbalism, homeopathy and acupuncture. In most member states of the EU, including Belgium, France, Spain, Italy and Greece, it is illegal for anyone except statutorily recognised health professionals to practise medicine; this includes all non-medically qualified complementary practitioners. However, in the Netherlands the government has stated that it will not prosecute non-medically qualified practitioners unless malpractice has been proved; complementary therapies are generally tolerated by the authorities and in fact flourish. In France and Spain, however, the authorities are particularly tough on clamping down on complementary practitioners. If measures in Paul Lannoye's report were adopted, practitioners would have the right to establish themselves anywhere in Europe, and all European citizens could have access to a wider choice of treatment options. In Germany the unique *Heilpraktiker* (health system) was introduced in 1939. It licenses practitioners who are not members of recognised health professions to practise complementary medicine provided they have passed an examination in basic medical knowledge and are registered.

But the wheels of Brussels grind slowly. Even if the Environment Committee and the Parliament vote for the Lannoye recommendations, they will not become law, but the move will open the door for future legislation on non-conventional medical disciplines.

Legislation governing complementary therapies in the UK

The practice of medicine is regulated by various Acts passed since the time of the Tudors and Stuarts. The Medical Act 1512 was the first to attempt to regulate the profession; it became an 'offence to practise physic or surgery' unless the practitioner was a university graduate or had been licensed by the bishop of the diocese in which he lived. This legislation was not popular, and as a result of public opinion the king was forced to amend the Act in 1542 to allow anyone to practise. This has become known as the Herbalists' Charter.

The Herbalists' Charter

This Act, which had the support of Henry VIII, was designed to help those people who could not afford the increasingly avaricious surgeons and physicians who allowed the sick 'to rot and perish to death' unless they could pay.

The legislation made it lawful for anyone who had knowledge and experience of the nature of 'Herbs, roots and Waters . . . to practise, use and minister in and to any outward sore, uncome, wound, apostemations, outward swelling or disease, any herb or herbs, oyntments, baths, pultres and amplaisters, according to their cunning, experience and knowledge . . . without suit, vexation, trouble, penalty, or loss of their goods'.

This right to practise freely and legally is guarded jealously by herbalists and supported by the government. Herbalists are under no obligation to clear what they prescribe with the Medicines Control Agency (the government regulatory body for medicines) – a privilege that they have had since Henry VIII's day, and which is much prized by them. Four hundred years later the Herbal Remedies Order 1977 defined the circumstances under which herbalists could prescribe certain toxic herbs, such as belladonna.

The Medical Act 1858

The Medical Act 1858 made it illegal for anyone who had not been registered as a qualified medical practitioner to claim to be one. It empowered the GMC to oversee the regulation and training of the profession. It did not prohibit non-orthodox or non-registered practitioners from treating patients, providing they did not claim to be registered doctors.

When it was first drafted, the Act contained a provision for any doctor who practised 'unconventional' forms of therapy to be struck off. This was rejected by both Houses of Parliament, and the final Act allowed doctors to use any form of treatment they chose, subject only to regulation by the GMC.

The Medicines Act 1968

Although the practitioners who dispense herbal and homeopathic remedies are not subject to regulation, the products they dispense are – at least in theory. Herbal goods manufactured in Britain are subject to statutory control, but imported and some mail-order products, used as stimulants, aphrodisiacs and tranquillisers, frequently evade it.

Both herbal and homeopathic preparations are subject to this Act, which deals with all medicinal products. Herbal remedies which did not have a licence before 1968 are exempted from licensing procedures. This exemption came under threat as a result of a EU directive in 1995 which required 'industrially produced medicinal products' to have a licence. After fierce lobbying from the herbalist and natural medicines movement the government introduced the Medicines for Human Use Regulations (Marketing Authorisations Etc.) in 1994.

Unlicensed preparations are thought to account for 80 per cent of all herbal sales. Many medicine-like products on the British market remain unregistered for two reasons: lack of sufficient acceptable data on their efficacy, safety and quality; and the high cost of the licensing fee.

Herbal products are made from well-known European herbs as well as less familiar Asian and South American ones, and from herbs with high safety records but also from those which may be contaminated with fungus, heavy metals, drugs or contain toxic plants, such as broom.

Under Section 12 of the Medicines Act 1968, herbal medicines which are manufactured, sold or supplied by someone in a face-to-face transaction do not have to be licensed. A herbalist does not have to list the ingredients in any remedy he or she prescribes. The product's safety and efficacy are the responsibility of the herbalist.

Special licensing procedures are already in place in Germany and France. Australia has developed an integrated approach to the herbal market which also covers non-Western herbs. Key elements of the Australian system include the need for compliance with codes of good manufacturing practice, lists of eligible herbs, and directions on labelling and claims made for the product.

How to complain about complementary practitioners

In a *Health Which?* survey published in December 1995, 85 out of 2,635 people who had visited a complementary practitioner said they had had a bad experience and wanted to complain. Thirty-three said they would have been satisfied with an apology.

If you feel you have been short-changed, either financially or in terms of the treatment you have received, you can do one or several of the following.

- Complain first directly to the practitioner. Talk or write to him or her about what happened (keep a copy of the letter). It may be that you have experienced a temporary adverse reaction commonly occurring after the type of treatment you have undergone.
- If you get no response from the practitioner and you want to take the matter further, complain in writing to the professional or regulatory body, such as the British Acupuncture Council, of which he is a member. Most have complaints procedures and codes of practice and ethics. The practitioner will usually be invited to respond, and a committee will decide what action should be taken.
- Complain in writing to the umbrella organisation, such as the BCMA or ICM, to which the therapist belongs. These bodies also have codes of conduct and can deal with complaints.
- If the practitioner is employed in a health centre or sports centre, complain in writing to its manager.
- If the practitioner is employed by the NHS and you see him on an NHS basis, you can use the NHS complaints procedure. If you have been referred to a complementary practitioner by your doctor under the NHS and are not happy with the treatment you have received, you should in the first instance complain to the practitioner, then to your GP; if you subsequently feel you have not received a satisfactory reply or explanation, complain to the senior partner in the GP practice.

HOW TO COMPLAIN ABOUT COMPLEMENTARY PRACTITIONERS

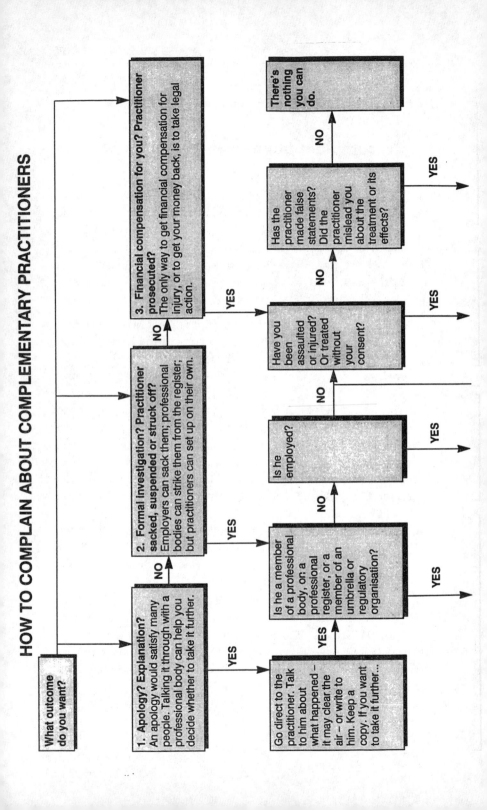

What outcome do you want?

1. Apology? Explanation? An apology would satisfy many people. Talking it through with a professional body can help you decide whether to take it further.

NO →

2. Formal investigation? Practitioner sacked, suspended or struck off? Employers can sack them; professional bodies can strike them from the register; but practitioners can set up on their own.

NO →

3. Financial compensation for you? Practitioner prosecuted? The only way to get financial compensation for injury, or to get your money back, is to take legal action.

YES ↓

Go direct to the practitioner. Talk to him about what happened – it may clear the air – or write to him. Keep a copy. If you want to take it further...

YES →

Is he a member of a professional body, on a professional register, or a member of an umbrella or regulatory organisation?

NO →

Is he employed?

YES →

NO →

Have you been assaulted or injured? Or treated without your consent?

YES →

NO →

Has the practitioner made false statements? Did the practitioner mislead you about the treatment or its effects?

YES →

NO →

There's nothing you can do.

Complain in writing to any relevant body:

Professional organisations: standards vary
The practitioner's letterhead or professional body or business card should tell you which register or professional bodies he or she belongs to (he may belong to several, or to none). The best have complaints procedures, and codes of practice and ethics. The practitioner will usually be invited to put his side and a committee will decide on action.

Umbrella organisations: a second chance of redress
The British Complementary Medicine Association and the Institute for Complementary Medicine have members in many different therapy areas. They also have codes of conduct and can deal with complaints.

Regulatory bodies: the best bet – where they exist
These set the standards for a profession. Membership of some is voluntary (e.g. British Acupuncture Council, Aromatherapy Organisations Council); others have legal powers (General Medical Council for doctors). The soon to be formed General Chiropractic Council and General Osteopathic Council will have legal status.

Complain to the employer
If the practitioner is employed, for example in a sports centre, beauty salon or complementary health centre, complain to the manager of the centre or salon.

Complain to the NHS
If you see the practitioner on the NHS, you can use NHS complaints procedures. For advice, contact the Health Information Line ✆ 0800 66544, or your local community health council, local health council in Scotland, or health and social services board in Northern Ireland (see the phone book).

LEGAL ACTION

Contact the police
Treating you without consent is assault in legal terms. But only the police can start a prosecution for criminal assault. And you won't necessarily be compensated.

Talk to an experienced solicitor
To get compensation, you may have to prove negligence, or that you have been assaulted if you didn't give consent. But it's vital to get advice from a lawyer who knows the area. Action for Victims of Medical Accidents can put you in touch with an expert solicitor. The Law Society may also be able to give you contacts.

Criminal prosecution
Under trade descriptions law, practitioners must not make false statements about their service or the effects of treatment. If they do, they can be prosecuted. You won't necessarily get any redress. Contact your local authority's trading standards department.

If you were misled...
If you can prove the practitioner misled you on the nature or effects of the treatment, you may be able to sue for compensation to cover your losses. It's likely to be time-consuming and costly; there's no guarantee of results. Talk first to an expert solicitor (see left). Using the small claims court will limit your costs.

Is the practitioner employed?

AND

YES

NO

Doctors cannot 'refer' you to a complementary practitioner in the same way that they can refer you to a hospital consultant. When a doctor refers you to another specialist, that specialist takes responsibility for your treatment – and takes the blame if anything goes wrong.

GPs 'delegate' your treatment to a complementary practitioner and remain responsible for the negligence of any complementary practitioner who is employed on a sessional basis, just as they do with non-clinical employees, such as receptionists.

If you had treatment under the NHS in a hospital which you consider unsatisfactory, complain in writing to the chief executive; your letter will be passed on to the complaints or customer services manager.

Your position if there is no improvement in your health

If you fail to get better after your treatment, theoretically you have no redress under the law; you have made the decision to trust and accept the professional judgement of a therapist, who may or may not be properly trained. If the therapy does not work, it is up to you to go elsewhere.

But at the same time, the practitioner is contracted to give you a service. You are paying money for this, possibly over a long period of time, and this is a contract. If you feel that the practitioner has not given you the agreed service, you can sue under the law of tort, as the practitioner has failed in his duty of care. Judges take a dim view of professionals who promise a specific service and fail to deliver.

Litigation

Despite the fact that complementary therapists are unregulated, they have a legal duty of care towards their patients, the breach of which could give rise to an allegation of negligence. If you have suffered personal injury at the hands of a complementary practitioner you have three years from the date of the accident or event in which to start legal action. If, however, there has been a breach of contract, whereby the service provided was defective but you did not suffer any injury, you would have six years in which to sue.

If the incident happened when you were a child or teenager, you have until you are 21 to bring an action.

On the basis of anecdotal evidence, it appears that cases of negligence against complementary practitioners are increasing, but the numbers that come to court are negligible. About 2 per cent of all claims brought against the NHS for medical negligence reach trial. The rest evaporate either because the claimant's expert says there is no case, or because the plaintiff, or victim, withdraws, or because there is an out-of-court settlement.

There are three reasons why people are reluctant to go to a lawyer after they have received bad treatment from a complementary practitioner: the fear of the legal costs involved; ignorance of their rights; and inertia.

In addition, so little has been written about what is right and what is not right in terms of treatment and how you should feel afterwards in the different spheres of complementary medicine that you may not be sure whether what happened to you is acceptable or not. The legal standard of care is a duty to act in accordance with a practice accepted as proper by a responsible body of professional opinion. In the absence of nationally agreed standards and qualifications in most therapies, it may be almost impossible to define what constitutes a reasonable standard of care.

If you have had a bad experience and think you might have a good case, first you must decide whom to sue. If your GP referred you to a complementary therapist, and you subsequently fell ill or incurred personal injury, you can sue both the therapist and the doctor. You will need professional advice, though: this is not a matter on which you should contemplate representing yourself in court (appearing as a litigant in person) or doing without legal help.

How to find a solicitor
It is best to go to a firm of solicitors which specialises in medical negligence cases and in plaintiff work. The Medical Negligence Panel of the Law Society* has 97 specialists on its books, and Action for Victims of Medical Accidents (AVMA)* has over 100. Such solicitors will know immediately to which expert the papers should be sent, what evidence to look for and how to get hold of your notes from your practitioner.

AVMA, which will give advice over the phone, produces an excellent booklet, *Medical Accidents*, containing explanations of how to complain and how to mount a legal action. You could also ring the Law Society Accident Line;* a receptionist will answer your call and ask you what your case is about. You will be given the telephone numbers of three solicitors in your area who deal with accidents. The solicitor will then give you a free consultation of 30 minutes.

Alternatively, your local Law Society or the Citizens Advice Bureau will put you in touch with an appropriate firm of solicitors. Your local library should hold a copy of the *Solicitors' Regional Directory*, which will list the names of specialised firms.

Are you eligible for legal aid?

If you are making a claim for financial compensation you would bring a civil action. You will be eligible for legal assistance under the 'green form scheme', which entitles you to some initial free legal advice, if your *disposable* income (that is, after tax, National Insurance and providing for your family and dependants) is £75 per week or less. If your income is higher you will not qualify. Whether or not you qualify for civil legal aid (i.e. full-blown legal aid) depends on your financial circumstances and the merits of your case. If you do, allowances are made for expenses such as rent or mortgage, but your disposable income must be no more than £7,403 a year.

Your capital must be below £1,000, plus dependants' allowances, for help under the green form scheme and below £6,750 for civil legal aid.

If you have legal aid and you lose your case, unless the Legal Aid Board* has ruled that you have to make a contribution, you need not pay any money to the defendant, i.e. the practitioner. The Legal Aid Board would pay the claimant's own expenses, and the practitioner would pay his own expenses. You can get information and booklets from the Press and Publications Section of the Legal Aid Board.

Who else might be able to help with legal fees?

If you are not eligible for legal aid, you may be covered for legal expenses under your household contents insurance. Some 10 per cent of people in the UK have some form of legal expenses insurance. It is an added extra in these policies, and many people forget that they have this cover or assume that the incident for which they are hiring a solicitor would not be covered by any insurance policy that they might hold.

Most insurance companies offer legal expenses cover and it costs only £5-£10 a year, so it is well worth having. It covers litigation concerning anything to do with your home, such as a dispute with your neighbour, and it also covers personal injury. If you are in any way injured by a complementary or medical practitioner, your insurance company may well pay your legal bill, usually up to £50,000, and sometimes more.

If you belong to a trade union it, too, may help. Many unions have arrangements with firms of solicitors and may fund an initial consultation with a solicitor or pay your legal fees up to an agreed level. But it is highly unlikely that a union will pay all your legal costs if the problem did not directly arise from your employment.

A firm of solicitors might agree to take your case on what is known as a 'conditional fee arrangement', that is, a 'no win, no fee' basis. Following the Courts and Legal Services Act 1990, since July 1995 solicitors have been allowed to offer conditional fee arrangements in England and Wales in the following types of cases: personal injury claims; certain bankruptcy/insolvency-related proceedings; and human rights cases (a similar system has been available in Scotland for some time). However, you must remember that although you would not have to pay your own solicitor's fees if you lost, you would still have to pay counsel's fees etc. and your opponent's costs (for a relatively small insurance premium you can insure against having to pay your opponent's legal costs). You must also be aware that because the 'no win, no fee' system is risky for the lawyer, he will agree with you an 'uplift' on his bill; this means that although you will pay him nothing if you lose, if you win you will have to pay his bill in full as well as an additional amount (agreed beforehand) for winning the case, which could be anything up to 100 per cent more than the original bill. Shop around as different lawyers will agree different 'uplift' levels.

Bringing a case in the small claims court
You could bring an action in the county court under the small claims procedure if the value of your claim is £3,000 or less. A typical claim in mainstream practice might be for having sustained a

minor eye injury in the course of having new contact lenses fitted at the opticians and being forced to take a week off work as a result.

For such actions you do not have to have legal representation and you do not have to have evidence from an expert. To instigate such a case, you should visit your local county court, explain that you want to proceed with such a claim, and the court clerk will give you the forms to fill in and help you to do so.

You will have to give a brief description of the injury and explain what financial losses you have incurred. If you are unable to drive, you could ask for travelling expenses; you may feel you need to be compensated for pain and suffering; if you are self-employed, you may lose work and want compensation for this.

The court would then start the process of bringing the action and serve papers on the practitioner at no expense to yourself. District judges, who sit in small claims courts, often rely on the evidence of the claimant alone as to the level of pain or injury.

'Consent' in medical practice

Common law recognises the principle that everyone has the right to have his or her bodily integrity respected. You should not be exposed to risk unless you have voluntarily accepted it on the basis of adequate information and understanding. Under the law you have sovereignty over what should happen to your body, and the law will protect you and your body from untoward interference.

Before any practitioner prescribes any medication or applies any form of lotion or substance or lays a hand on your body, it is vital that he ensures that you are aware of what is going to happen, what the nature of the treatment might be and what risks might flow from it; all of this should be discussed before treatment begins.

Lack of communication and a failure to inform you about what is going to happen is more likely to happen in mainstream medicine; most complementary practitioners are very good at telling their clients what they are going to do.

If there is a breach of this law of consent – in other words, something happened to you which you did not expect and to which you had not agreed – there are two options open to you:

●   you can claim for damages for **failure to warn**. This will be a civil action and usually comes under negligence

- you can bring a charge of **battery and assault** under Section 39 of the Criminal Justice Act 1988. An **assault** is committed 'when the defendant intentionally or recklessly causes his victim to apprehend the immediate infliction of unlawful force'. It is sufficient in law if the victim anticipated violence. **Battery** is committed when the defendant 'intentionally or recklessly inflicts unlawful force'. A battery may follow an assault. The slightest touching, if unlawful, may be sufficient to amount to battery. In one case (Lord Lane C.J. Faulkner *v* Talbot 1981) it was ruled that battery was 'any intentional touching of another person without the consent of that person and without lawful excuse. It need not necessarily be hostile, rude, or aggressive.' Assault and battery are summary offences, tried in a magistrates' court with maximum penalties of six months' imprisonment or a fine, or both. Where the violent act amounts to a criminal offence, you may obtain damages through the Criminal Injuries Compensation Scheme, or alternatively pursue a claim for personal injury through the civil court. It would be advisable to contact the police, especially if you wish to bring a prosecution for criminal assault.

Anyone suffering a personal injury may bring a claim for compensation and damages against the person who caused the injury. Physical injury includes psychological damage, provided that the damage is a recognised psychological condition (the most obvious example is post-traumatic stress disorder).

If you are physically injured as a result of a treatment or feel that the practitioner breached the legal duty of care to which he is bound, you may have a civil claim for negligence against the practitioner under medical law.

A typical case might be someone with a history of back pain who visited an osteopath or chiropractor, perhaps for the first time, and after one treatment noticed a marked increase in pain. The client might attribute the increase in pain to the manipulation that took place on that date.

In order to establish negligence, you would have to prove that the practitioner owed you a duty of care and that he was in breach of that duty of care. Any practitioner who enters a therapeutic relationship with a patient – whether the medicine he practises is mainstream or complementary – is under a duty not to harm that person. You must also prove that you suffered injury.

Even if the practitioner was negligent, it has to be proved that the technique that day actually caused the injury; it may well be that the injury was caused by something else.

The knottiest problem in proving negligence is the second point – whether the practitioner gave you the appropriate standard of care; this is the standard of care exercised by a reasonable person professing to have those skills. If the practitioner conducted his treatment in a way that any reasonable person with those skills would have conducted it, then your case for negligence would collapse.

The standard test case for medical negligence was that of Bolam *v* Friern Hospital Management Committee. In broad terms, this established that if the actions of the practitioner fall within the area of treatment that would have been performed by a responsible body of practitioners in that particular art, then no negligence would be found by the court. If a technique can be carried out in ten different ways and the court finds that a third of 'reasonable' practitioners in that specific field would have done the same thing in the same circumstances, then the court would find that practitioner was not negligent.

It is therefore vital, before you start on the long and expensive road of litigation, to make sure that you have a case. For that an expert is needed, who can tell you and your solicitor whether the treatment received fell outside the treatment that would be considered normal. If your case is in any way weak, the defendant's expert witness will pick up on it.

After your initial consultation with your solicitor, which could last well over an hour, the solicitor will try to obtain the notes and records that the practitioner kept of your visit.

Three statutes grant specific rights of access to health information – the Data Protection Act 1984, the Access to Medical Reports 1988 and the Access to Health Records Act 1990. These have all been amended to include osteopaths and chiropractors, but the patient has a statutory right of access only to medical records held by 'health professionals' as defined in Section 2 of the Access to Health Records Act.

This is subject to the Data Protection Act, which provides for an individual's right to see personal data about him which is held on computer. There can be no justification for a practitioner to withhold any patient's notes. Most notes are obtained under what is called 'pre-action discovery' under Section 3A of the Supreme Court Act 1981.

If the practitioner is loath to release them, it can take some time. It might even be necessary to obtain a court order, which involves expense, to force the practitioner to release them; but this is most unlikely. The solicitor will then take a look at the documents to see if there is a case for a claim or not. The papers will then be referred to an expert for a full report as to whether there is liability or not. An expert's report can cost anything from £300 to £1,000 depending on the amount of paperwork involved, and whether or not he will need to examine you. If the expert believes the case is not strong enough for a claim, it will go no further. The lawyer will not proceed and you would be left with a hefty legal bill (to cover the cost of sending the papers to an expert, for example), which could be anything from £500 to £2,000.

Product liability

The Consumer Protection Act 1987 applies to unsafe or defective products. Under the terms of the Act, a product is considered defective if 'the safety of the product is not such as persons generally are entitled to expect'. Under product liability legislation you can sue the manufacturer, the importer and the shop where you bought it.

However, the onus is on you to show that the product is defective. The lotion that you were given by the practitioner or bought off the shelf may well have given you a rash, but if when analysed it is found to be harmless, you will have no case.

Other legislation which may be useful is the Trades Description Act 1968 and health and safety laws such as the Health and Safety at Work Act 1974. The Control of Substances Hazardous to Health (COSHH) Regulations 1988 deal with hazardous chemicals and body fluids which may be infectious. An acupuncturist using unsterilised needles would be liable under this legislation.

Is legal action the right course to take?

Legal action can be a long, harrowing and expensive process. It can take two years or longer, and although your solicitor will do most of the work you will be expected to take an active interest and will have to deal with letters and attend meetings. You may have to be examined by a doctor or therapist acting either for you or for the practitioner concerned.

Nevertheless, if you have the right solicitor, a strong case and the support of your family and friends, and are fully aware of the problems that may arise, you should not be dissuaded from taking legal action.

PART II

A–Z OF COMPLEMENTARY THERAPIES

ACUPUNCTURE

IN A survey published in *Which?* in November 1995 (see Appendix), acupuncture was the fourth most popular therapy after osteopathy, chiropractic and homeopathy. The survey also showed that 80 per cent of respondents who had undergone acupuncture in the previous 12 months were satisfied with the treatment they had received.

Doctors are beginning to pay closer attention to acupuncture. It is used in all pain clinics and in some maternity units to alleviate pain. Patients undergoing chemotherapy have also been treated with acupuncture to lessen the discomfort caused by vomiting and nausea.

The two main types of acupuncture practised in Britain are traditional Chinese acupuncture, which works on the meridian principle and balancing energy; and medical acupuncture, sometimes called Western or scientific acupuncture. Medical acupuncture is practised by doctors who have had supplementary training in acupuncture and use the therapy in addition to their orthodox treatments. Some medical acupuncturists are also traditional acupuncturists. In addition to the 1,400 members on the register of the British Acupuncture Council,* over 1,400 doctors have been trained and registered with the British Medical Acupuncture Society.* Some work as anaesthetists, but 70 per cent are GPs offering acupuncture as part of their NHS practices.

The theory behind it

Acupuncture is one of the principal components of traditional Chinese medicine, which also encompasses herbal medicine, diet, massage, acupressure, manipulative therapy, relaxation and special exercises. In Chinese medicine, the body is thought to possess a network of invisible pathways called meridians. Along these meridians flows a life-energy or *qi* (pronounced 'chee') comprising balanced components called *yin* and *yang*. These components are not substances, but two opposites, which exist in nature and should be in balance. *Yin* is associated with darkness, rest, earth, matter, inwardness, downwardness, femaleness and water; *yang* is light, activity, heaven, energy, expansion, rising, maleness and fire. When the *qi* becomes deficient, blocked or 'stagnant' or when the *yin* and *yang* become unbalanced, the theory goes, illness results.

Acupuncturists aim to restore the balance of energy in the body by freeing or unblocking the meridians by placing needles in specific points along them. The needles can be used to stimulate or boost *qi*, to disperse or unblock it or just to activate a point. Chinese medicine recognises 12 paired main meridians (corresponding to each of the five *yin* and six *yang* organs and to the pericardium), one posterior and one anterior channel, and 365 acupoints along them. It has been suggested that there are as many as 500 points, but most acupuncturists use something like 150 or more in their everyday practice. One of the main tasks of the acupuncturist is to observe the relationship between *yin* and *yang* in the body and make adjustments to bring about harmony, or *tao*. A person can have an excess of fire, heat, dryness or be hyperactive, in which case he will have too much *yang*; or he could have too much water, cold, wet and be lethargic (*yin*).

The forces of *yin* and *yang* are in balance in a healthy person, allowing the *qi* to flow freely through the meridians, each of which is associated with different organs (which do not correspond to Western anatomical organs), or bodily functions. *Yin* meridians run from the toes or fingertips upwards, *yang* meridians run from the head to the fingertips or toes.

Qi takes 24 hours to flow round the body and each meridian has a time of the day when the *qi* is at its strongest. This might explain why some people are 'larks' (at their best in the early morning) and others 'owls' (at their best at night).

Qi might be a strange concept to Westerners, but the idea that living things have 'energy' or a 'life force' is recognised in several other cultures. In Japan the force is called *ki*, in India it is known as *prana,* in Tibet, it is *rlun*. *Qi* is simply that which makes us alive.

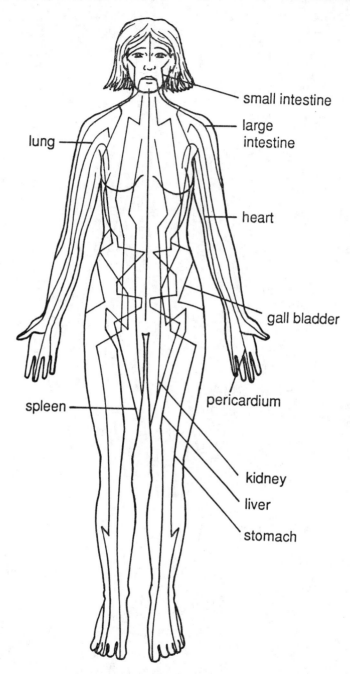

small intestine

large intestine

lung

heart

gall bladder

pericardium

spleen

kidney

liver

stomach

Figure 1 Main meridian lines on the front of the body

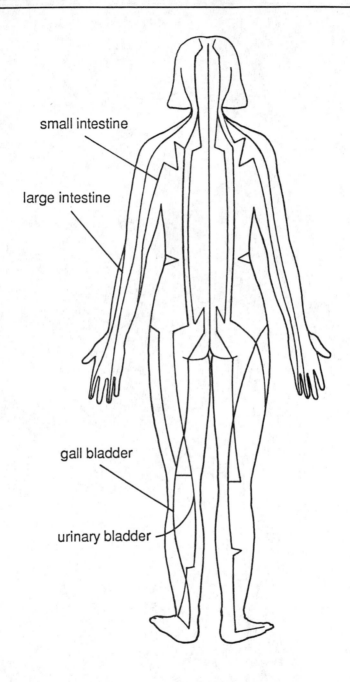

Figure 2 Main meridian lines on the back of the body

One explanation of how acupuncture works is that a nerve impulse is fired off to the spinal cord from the needle insertion. This in turn releases the body's natural painkiller, endorphins. Another is based on the 'gate' theory of pain which claims that pain impulses can be regulated by a 'gate' along the pathways of the nervous system and that certain nerve fibres, stimulated by acupuncture, close this gate and shut off the pain.

Some people also believe that acupuncture causes the release of three neurotransmitters in the brain, which have the effect of making you feel drowsy and relaxed and have an impact on the body's hormones, which in turn can have a beneficial effect. It is also thought to influence the limbic centre in the brain which controls mood and behaviour – and an area which is thought to be concerned with addiction.

What it might be good for

Acupuncture has often been used for pain relief. However, it can be used to treat almost anything that you would go to your GP for, including back pain, migraine, menstrual problems, menopausal symptoms, joint pain and arthritis, backache, high blood pressure, insomnia and cystitis. It can also be used for pain relief in childbirth.

It has been used to treat the nausea caused by chemotherapy and is increasingly being incorporated into drug detoxification programmes. Some practitioners treat people who are HIV-positive.

Practitioners also claim that it can alleviate emotional problems (anxiety, stress, depression), respiratory ailments (sinusitis, hay fever) and digestive disorders such as irritable bowel syndrome. Acupuncture has been used successfully with the terminally ill, not because it can cure them but because it works on the emotions and spirit. Acupuncturists who work with those in this situation say that the therapy helps their patients to deal with the diagnosis and make their peace with the world.

History

Acupuncture is a Chinese method of treatment that goes back at least 2,000 years. Cave paintings in China depict what look like acupuncture needles.

Legend has it that acupuncture was discovered when physicians attending battlefields saw soldiers with arrow wounds cured of old injuries or chronic ailments. The physicians took note of precisely where the wounds were and then began to experiment by sticking fishbones and flakes of flint into specific areas of the body. The first medical textbook on the subject, the *Huang-di Nei-jing* (*Inner Classic of the Yellow Emperor*), was published between 300 and 100 BC. This has been called the bible of Chinese medicine.

Acupuncture was brought to Europe in the nineteenth century by missionaries and other people returning from the colonies. However, the techniques taken up by early Western 'acupuncturists' were fairly heavy-handed and it fell into disrepute.

It was revived in the 1930s by a French diplomat, Georges Soulie de Morant, who had worked in China. He published an acupuncture manual, *A Summary of the True Art of Chinese Acupuncture*. By the 1960s a few articles had appeared in the national press about it, but it was not until Richard Nixon's trip to China in 1972 that the West began to take serious notice.

Today between 5 and 10 per cent of anaesthetic procedures in China use electro-acupuncture and the patients usually receive a painkiller and sedative as well. It is never used for emergency surgery.

Treatment

If you visit a traditional acupuncturist, your first session will take about an hour. As for all types of Oriental medicine, diagnosis involves four elements: asking, observing, listening and touching. The practitioner will ask you about and take detailed notes of your signs and symptoms, medical history, family history, lifestyle and diet, and will want to know whether your bowels work regularly, whether you sleep well, and your reactions to stress, heat and cold. He or she will ask you many of the usual questions your GP might ask, but also things like 'Do you feel cold?' or 'How do you feel about sadness?'.

Acupuncturists, like practitioners of other Chinese therapies, do not use X-rays or blood tests. In addition to the information they obtain from the patient, they rely on their senses of sight and smell for diagnostic information. The practitioner will therefore observe your posture, the way you walk and sit, and the shine in your eyes and hair, and listen to what your voice sounds like.

The touching element of the diagnosis involves taking the pulse and palpating the abdomen. Your pulse will be taken at both wrists. There are six pulses in each wrist and they can have up to 28 qualities including wiry, empty, floating, rapid, slippery, knotted and intermittent. Feeling the pulse is regarded as one of the most important parts of diagnosis in traditional Chinese medicine, and textbooks list more than 32 abnormal pulses – including a 'floating' pulse which can be felt only with a light touch, a 'deep' pulse which can hardly be felt by a light touch and a 'rapid' pulse. The practitioner will also gently palpate your abdomen to assess the energy flow in the meridians and internal organs.

Your tongue will most certainly be examined; in traditional Chinese medicine this is an important part of the diagnosis. If you are healthy your tongue should be pink, moist and with a thin white coating. The therapist will look to see if the tongue is swollen, pale or red, or furry – all of which indicate certain conditions.

Once you have been diagnosed, you may be asked to undress partially (not always, as this depends on where the practitioner chooses to place the needles) and to lie on a couch. The acupuncturist will then place the needles in certain points along chosen meridians. The most commonly used points are along the limbs, below the knees and between the elbows and the fingers.

The needles are usually made of stainless steel and are almost as fine as a hair. When they are inserted there is often little or no pain, although some people find them uncomfortable and others feel a strange, dull ache or pulling sensation deeper in the limb. This, according to practitioners, is the needle gripping the qi. It is the feeling that acupuncturists want – a sign that they have located the qi. However, if you do not feel it, it does not mean the treatment is not working. Acupuncturists say a successfully inserted needle feels as if it is going into something, as if it has been grabbed by the energy; if it misses the point it feels as if it is going into nothing. Needles are usually inserted to a depth of a centimetre, but they can go as deep as 12 cm, depending on which part of the body the acupuncturist is treating. At the nail point, for example, the needles would go in a millimetre; in the buttocks the depth could be several centimetres. They are left in place for up to 20 minutes or occasionally longer. Sometimes the acupuncturist will manipulate the needles periodically between the thumb and first finger, and this can feel uncomfortable.

The acupuncturist may well use other traditional Chinese medicine therapies. You may have moxibustion, derived from the Japanese word *moekusa,* meaning 'burning herb'. The aim of moxibustion is to warm the *qi.* The practitioner places a small cone of the powdered leaves of a herb, usually mugwort, over an acupuncture point either at the end of a needle or close to the skin. It is allowed to burn so that the patient can feel heat, but not so that it burns the skin. This is repeated several times on the same point. Sometimes a slice of garlic or ginger is sandwiched between the cone and the skin.

Another method is to ignite the tip of a cigar-shaped 'moxa' stick and place it a few centimetres away from the skin over the acupuncture point. The acupuncturist may also use 'cupping' – placing cups on the skin at strategic points.

Some, but not all, acupuncturists may recommend herbs or herbal pills (see Chinese herbal medicine) and others may use acupressure (massage on acupuncture points). This is used mainly in situations where it may be difficult or dangerous to use acupuncture or moxibustion.

Electrical stimulation is sometimes used with acupuncture. Once the acupuncturist has inserted the needles they are connected to a battery-operated electrical device which produces a tingling sensation which is not uncomfortable.

Some people feel energised after an acupuncture treatment; some feel sleepy and relaxed. The points where the needles were inserted may be a bit tender for a couple of hours. Most people sleep well the night after a treatment.

How often you should visit an acupuncturist will depend on your condition. Some people go for acupuncture treatment occasionally, just to keep healthy; others go with a specific ailment. Usually people start off with a course of three to six sessions, and at the end of that time the practitioner reviews the situation. You will usually need several sessions to begin to feel real benefit.

Does it work?

Anecdotal evidence that acupuncture works is strong. Plenty of individual reports have been written in support of it, and there have been over 700 randomised trials of the therapy.

Studies have tended to be fairly small, but slowly scientific research is beginning to match anecdotal evidence. In one study in Scandinavia, researchers found an 80 per cent reduction in pain in 29 patients with severe knee osteoarthritis waiting for surgery; seven patients decided after their treatment that they did not want the operation.

There is some evidence that acupuncture may be able to benefit some of Britain's 3 million asthma sufferers. Other studies show that acupuncture is effective in reducing nausea linked to surgery, pregnancy and chemotherapy. See Chapter 3 for details of more scientific research.

Can it do any harm?

It is often taken for granted that acupuncture is essentially harmless and indeed it has often been asserted that it is totally safe. This claim is not true. A study published in 1996 in Norway showed that pneumothorax (puncturing of the lung), fainting during acupuncture and increased pain after the treatment may be more common than previously thought.

The Norwegian researchers surveyed 1,135 doctors trained in acupuncture and 197 acupuncturists, asking them about adverse effects of acupuncture. Just over a third of the acupuncturists and 12 per cent of the doctors reported adverse effects from acupuncture treatment including local skin infections and lungs punctured by acupuncture needles.

Unsterilised needles can transmit infections, including hepatitis and the HIV virus. Qualified acupuncturists can, however, be relied upon to use needles that are either sterilised or sealed in sterile packets and disposable, so the risk of infection should be minute.

In the Norwegian study, 132 patients fainted during treatment and the respondents cited a total of 33 cases of pneumothorax. Many reports of pneumothorax as a result of acupuncture have been made throughout the world.

Other problems include damaged tissues (and even organs if the needles are inserted too deeply or at the wrong site). Parts of acupuncture needles have been found in patients' kidneys, spines, spinal cords and hearts, according to one study.

In 1995 a review was undertaken of all the available literature: over 100 papers reported complications as a result of acupuncture, of which there were a total of 395 cases of adverse effects. Many of the reports were anecdotal.

This may sound alarming if you are considering whether or not to have acupuncture, but it is important to keep things in perspective. In all, only 216 instances of *serious* complications worldwide over a 20-year period have been reported. Bearing in mind the thousands of consultations taking place in the UK alone every year, this figure is very low.

How to choose a practitioner

At the moment anyone (including doctors) can legally call him or herself an acupuncturist and start sticking needles into people, so it is important to check qualifications.

There are two major organisations in the field of acupuncture: the British Acupuncture Council (BAcC), which represents acupuncturists who are not medically qualified (they will carry MBAcC after their name), and the British Medical Acupuncture Society (BMAS), whose members are doctors of medicine.

The BAcC, launched in 1995, brought together Britain's five acupuncture bodies under one umbrella. Its goal is to move the profession towards state registration, in line with osteopaths and chiropractors. The BAcC holds a register of its members who follow a code of ethics and practice; those practising in the UK are covered by professional indemnity and insurance.

Acupuncturists belonging to the BAcC must have the equivalent of two years' full-time training, and that training must be similar to that which the British Acupuncture Accreditation Board (BAAB), which was set up by the BAcC, now stipulates.

The BMAS offers two levels of training to its members. The first level is the basic competence in acupuncture, which is studied over several weekends on top of the doctors' clinical training, and must include evidence of 30 case histories. Further specialist training is covered by the certificate of accreditation, for which the practitioner must have 100 hours' training in acupuncture, plus 100 case histories written up in a logbook, 20 of which must be in detail.

There is a certain rivalry between the two organisations. Some doctors in the BMAS hold that only medically qualified people should practise acupuncture. They maintain that non-medically qualified acupuncturists should not stick needles into people and may miss important signs and symptoms of serious illness. Traditional acupuncturists, on the other hand, frown on the short training that doctors have in a technique which in China takes between six and ten years to master. Fully qualified traditional acupuncturists say they can spot serious conditions and would then advise patients to see their GPs as necessary.

The real danger, however, lies with neither of these two groups, but with the 'practitioner' who sets up shop with little or no training (and may then charge exorbitant fees).

The acupuncturist's answers to the following questions will be useful in helping you make your choice:

- is he or she registered with a recommended registered body? is that body governed by a code of ethics and conduct and is there a lay person monitoring these codes?
- does the practitioner have liability insurance?
- how much will the treatment cost?
- how many sessions might your treatment require?

Cost

Between £15 and £40 per session, depending on where the practitioner is based, plus the cost of any herbs or herbal pills.

ALEXANDER TECHNIQUE

IN THE mid-1980s few people had heard of the Alexander technique. Now there are about 700 teachers (as practitioners prefer to be called) in the UK and it is rapidly increasing in popularity.

The theory behind it

The Alexander technique is not so much a therapy as a form of education. The practitioner teaches the pupil to develop more efficient postural behaviour through a series of lessons in which awareness of the body, posture and postural bad habits is enhanced.

The idea of 'use' is important to Alexander teachers. All activities – walking, sitting, reading, even talking – involve the use of many muscles. Most of us have postural bad habits, such as slouching, sagging, cocking our heads to the side, bending forwards from our waists when we walk and staring at the ground.

Many of these habits are picked up in childhood from watching the people around us, or from carrying heavy books to school. By the time we reach adulthood these habits have become part of us, and we are unaware of our poor posture. Many people think that is just how they are, as if posture were something we are born with. However, once postural harmony has been achieved, once we have learned to use our bodies correctly in everyday life, the body gains greater freedom, and functions such as breathing, circulation, digestion and bowel movements are made easier.

What it might be good for

Practitioners claim that Alexander technique is good for most musculo-skeletal disorders. The most common reasons why people opt for lessons in Alexander technique are lower back pain, chronic migraine or joint conditions such as arthritis. It is also said to benefit whiplash injuries, repetitive strain injury and stress-related conditions. Alexander teachers also claim it helps those with mental disorders such as depression.

It is also popular with actors, musicians and singers because it appears to benefit breathing, pre-performance 'nerves' and the voice. Several music colleges offer Alexander lessons: it can help ease sore fingers and joints (for instance, from piano- or violin-playing) and release tension from the muscles around the vocal cords. The Alexander technique has been part of a £2 million programme funded by the British Performing Arts Medicine Trust to deal with stage fright.

History

The Alexander technique was invented by an Australian actor, Frederick Matthias Alexander. He suffered from respiratory problems, and the stress of his profession affected his voice to such an extent that he could hardly finish one performance. Doctors told him to rest his voice, but this had little effect and on the night of his next performance his voice cracked again.

He began to suspect it was something he was doing that was affecting his voice. Watching himself in mirrors, he noticed that when he began to recite his part he drew in air sharply and tensed his neck muscles. This pulled his head back and down and compressed his vocal cords. By careful observation and experimentation, he devised a technique which cured his rasping voice. He discovered that efficiency in all activities depends on a balanced relationship between the head, neck and spine.

Treatment

The technique is very restful and calming. It is probably best to dress in leggings or a tracksuit, but this is not essential. During the first session, the teacher will probably ask you to walk around the room and sit down, to see how you use your body. The teacher will be interested in what type of work you do (whether manual or sedentary), but will not need to know about your personal life, unless it produces any stress which may affect your balance and posture.

Having observed you, the teacher may ask you to lie on a couch, with your head on a small pile of books and your knees raised. The teacher will use his or her hands gently to persuade your muscles to relax so that the limbs re-align themselves. The teacher will look at the way you sit and teach you how to sit down correctly, with back straight and head forward. When you rise, the head, neck and torso should move as one. Over a number of lessons, the teacher will draw attention to your posture, and explain how best to achieve a more natural one.

There is no tugging or pulling or thrusting; the teacher will gently lay his or her hands on various parts of your body. If, for example, you have a tendency to bend slightly at the knees when you stand, the teacher will not tell you to stand up straight or snap your knees back. You will be asked to concentrate on the muscles at the back of your knees, your ankles and around your neck and to imagine that the ankles and heels are rooted to the floor.

To begin with, you need the teacher to analyse your posture and balance, but later he or she will teach you techniques which you can apply to your everyday activities. One such exercise is to lie on the floor relaxed with a book under your head and the knees bent upwards for about 15 minutes. This will ease the lower back, but although it sounds easy, it is hard to achieve. Many people find it difficult to find the time or to rest the mind completely: in the therapy class they feel relaxed and completely free of stress.

Each lesson lasts about 45 minutes. You will usually have 'grown' by about 1 cm after the lesson, and, if you are driving, you will find you have to adjust your mirror.

Does it work?

Many people claim that the Alexander technique has unknotted them and freed their body from years of tension. They move better, their bodies lengthen and they walk more elegantly. Energy that used to be spent in unnecessary actions and movements is now put to better use.

The technique can also be used to ease pain. Pain causes stress which leads to muscle tension, which in turn leads to further pain. Alexander teachers claim the technique has a powerful impact on pain, releasing the muscles and freeing the body.

There have been a handful of controlled studies of the technique. Between 1955 and 1972 researchers at Tufts University, Boston, demonstrated changes in movement and muscle tension patterns after Alexander lessons. Another study in 1983, done at the Columbia-Presbyterian Medical Center, New York, showed that the breathing of patients undergoing tuition improved.

A study carried out in 1992 looked at the effects of Alexander technique on respiratory function. Ten healthy adult volunteers received 20 private lessons at weekly intervals. A further ten healthy volunteers, matched for age, sex, height and weight, acted as controls. The group receiving treatment showed significant increases in respiratory muscular strength and endurance. The researchers concluded that this was because the Alexander technique increased the length of the torso muscles.

Can it do any harm?

Because it is such a gentle technique, it causes no harm and is suitable for all ages.

How to choose a practitioner

Most doctors approve of the Alexander technique, so although you are extremely unlikely to receive it free on the NHS, your GP may recommend a local teacher. The main umbrella organisation in the UK is the Society of Teachers of the Alexander Technique,* whose members may be recognised by the initials MSTAT (Member of the Society of Teachers of the Alexander Technique).

The Society supervises training, upholds a code of ethics and maintains a register of teachers. All its members are insured and many attend the regular postgraduate and professional development courses the Society provides. About 65 Alexander teachers in the UK do not belong to STAT.

Success relies on building up a rapport with your teacher, so arrange a trial lesson to see whether you get on with the teacher and the technique.

Cost

About £25 per session. The technique is very unlikely to be available on the NHS, though the British Medical Association says referrals by GPs are 'occasional and increasing'. To make a real change STAT recommends a minimum of 20 lessons.

Aromatherapy

AROMATHERAPY may not be the most popular complementary therapy in Britain, but according to a Mintel report published in 1994 it is the fastest-growing. The sale of aromatherapy oils accounted for £10 million in 1994 and increased by almost 70 per cent between 1992 and 1994. In a *Which?* survey published in November 1995 (see Appendix), 12 per cent of respondents who had ever tried a complementary therapy said they had visited an aromatherapist in the previous year.

Aromatherapy is increasingly being used in health and beauty clinics and gyms. Nurses in hospitals and hospices use it to help alleviate sleep problems, pain and stress, not because they want to jump on the complementary bandwagon, but because they find it effective.

The theory behind it

Aromatherapy is based on the healing properties of essential plant oils. These oils are what gives rose petals their distinctive perfume, or a twig of rosemary its strong, woody smell. They are present in tiny droplets in the plant and are exuded in greater concentrations at certain times of the year and day or night. These oils readily evaporate: when you put your nose to a lily, it is the vapour from the essential oil that you are smelling.

Essential oils are extracted from the flowers, leaves, fruit, seeds and bark of certain plants by steam distillation. They have a highly complex chemical structure and each of the 400 plant essences that exist is said to have different characteristics – for instance, geranium and sage are believed to be stimulating, bergamot and lavender calming. The body 'activates' the oil by absorbing it into the skin.

The oils are usually massaged into the body, but they can be inhaled, used in a bath or in a cold compress next to the skin. The aim of aromatherapy is to support the body in its fight against disease.

There are three types of aromatherapy:

- holistic aromatherapy, which uses essential oils and massage to treat a range of emotional and physical disorders
- clinical aromatherapy, which integrates aromatherapy with orthodox treatments. Clinical aromatherapy is not advocated in the UK
- aesthetic aromatherapy, which is used by beauty therapists to relax clients and to treat some skin problems such as acne or stretch marks.

It is important not to confuse the three. Aesthetic aromatherapy is wonderfully relaxing and is used with great success not only as a beauty therapy but in residential homes for the elderly and in hospices. However, it is not a yardstick by which to judge the whole therapy.

What it might be good for

Because it encourages relaxation, aromatherapy is said to be good for stress-related conditions. Digestive problems respond well as do muscular aches and pains, premenstrual syndrome, painful periods and menopausal problems. Aromatherapists claim that it can also benefit skin conditions, such as eczema and rosacea (reddening of the skin).

In the *Which?* survey, of those who expressed an opinion about aromatherapy just over a quarter said they felt the treatment had greatly improved their condition and nine out of ten said they were 'satisfied' with the treatment.

History

Humans have a basic need for smell. The idea that we have somehow 'grown out' of this need because we are civilised was a mistake made by space scientists in the 1960s and early '70s. They sent their astronauts into space without anything pleasant to smell, except for lemon-scented hand-wipes. Before long, these wipes were not used for cleansing at all, but saved up for sniffing sessions. On later flights, the astronauts were provided with fragrances and bottled reproductions of familiar smells to remind them of home.

The distillation of essential oils began in the Middle East. The knowledge of how these oils can be used for healing was probably introduced to Europe by the Romans, although there is plenty of evidence that the inhabitants of Europe at the time used herbs for medicinal purposes.

Perfumes were in great demand in Europe in the sixteenth and seventeenth centuries. In 1597 a German physician, Heironymus Braunschweig, published a weighty tome listing 25 essential oils and their uses. Soon essential oils were being routinely stocked by herbalists.

In the eighteenth century essential oils were used by all herbalists and some doctors, but by the nineteenth century, with the rise of the 'orthodox' medical practitioners and the dwindling popularity of the herbalist, their use diminished. Herbalists themselves had less and less recourse to essential oils.

It was a French chemist, René-Maurice Gattefosse, who coined the term 'aromatherapy' in 1937. He made it the title of his book about the healing properties of oil. He was particularly interested in the use of oils for skin problems, recognising their value as antibacterial agents. He discovered, after burning his hand in a laboratory accident, the beneficial effect that lavender oil could have on a burn.

Gattefosse was not the only chemist to investigate the benefits of essential oils, but research ground to a halt during the Second World War. A French army surgeon, Dr Jean Valnet, used it to treat war wounds and published a book on the subject. The popularity and respectability accorded to aromatherapy in France have continued.

In Britain, aromatherapy was re-introduced by Robert Tisserand in 1969. He started the first training institute in the 1970s.

Treatment

First of all, before opting for aromatherapy make sure that this is a suitable therapy for you. If you have hypersensitive skin, and perfume brings you up in a rash, then you may not be able to tolerate essential oils either. Most perfume ingredients and essential oils have the potential to cause minor skin irritation.

The first session with an aromatherapist may be up to two hours long, during which the therapist will ask you about your medical history, your health, lifestyle, work and so on. He or she will select essential oils that are beneficial for you at that time. Subsequent sessions will last an hour.

A good aromatherapist will have a large selection of oils from which to choose. These will be mixed with a carrier oil, such as almond. Pure essential oil should never be applied to the skin. The blend of oils the aromatherapist prepares is designed to work on the physical, mental and 'subtle' energies of the body at the same time. The treatment will be smooth and slow, like a Swedish massage.

The massage itself will relax you, and often releases emotional as well as physical tension. Some people feel a little disoriented or light-headed afterwards, or simply relaxed. You will not reek of perfume – all of it will have been absorbed – neither will you be greasy for, again, all the oil will have been massaged in.

Some people may have a reaction, such as a headache, to aromatherapy and may feel worse, but this should not last for more than a couple of days and is usually followed by the opposite – a feeling of well-being. If you do have a reaction, it is wise to ring the aromatherapist.

Does it work?

Few randomised controlled clinical trials have been undertaken on aromatherapy and no research on whether its benefits are due to the relaxing massage or the oils themselves.

Essential oils stimulate the sense of smell, which in turn affects the area of the brain known as the limbic system. This is connected with instinctive behaviour, strong emotions and mood control. Walk into your old school five, ten or 20 years after you left it and you will probably pick up a distinctive smell that will conjure up long-buried feelings and memories. Experiments have been carried out on animals which show that clary-sage and ylang-ylang make dogs docile, while wormwood, hyssop and sage can make them aggressive.

The link between emotions – fear, love, excitement, anger – and the release of body chemicals is well established. Aromatherapy, through its impact on the limbic system, can stimulate the release of neurochemicals, as well as hormones, in the body.

Because of their tiny molecular structure essential oils can easily be absorbed through the skin into the bloodstream. Minute molecules of essential oil carried in the blood stream are believed to affect different organ functions. Since the turn of the century chemists have been publishing studies on essential oils, but most of them have been done *in vitro* in a laboratory. It is harder to test the impact of essential oils on the human body. There is mounting evidence, however, that essential oils have a role to play as antibiotics. Scientific studies have shown that many oils can fight bacteria directly. A study published in 1995 in France showed that tea-tree oil has an impact on methicillin-resistant *Staphylococcus aureus* (MRSA), a bacterium that is very much on the increase in hospitals.

Essential oils can relieve some of the symptoms of infection. *Eucalyptus globulus*, for instance, is a decongestant and therefore useful for respiratory problems. Both eucalyptus and lavender are highly sedative and calming.

The mental health organisation MIND says in its policy statement on treatments for depression that options apart from drugs should include 'alternatives such as massage, aromatherapy, herbal medicine, yoga' and medical staff have reported that aromatherapy seems to have a beneficial impact on depressed patients.

Elderly people can also benefit from aromatherapy. The Central and Cecil Housing Trust, which runs sheltered accommodation in west London, carried out a six-month study looking at the impact of various complementary therapies, including aromatherapy, among its residents (see Chapter 2). Researchers found that the therapies could relieve many of the classic symptoms of conditions common among the elderly – sleeplessness, anxiety, depression, arthritis and senile dementia. Aromatherapy was found to induce feelings of peace and pleasure, and one resident achieved her first full night's sleep in four years after regular aromatherapy. Many residents stopped or reduced their intake of painkillers and sedatives.

Dr Tim Betts, a consultant neuropsychiatrist at Queen Elizabeth Psychiatric Hospital in Birmingham, is successfully using essential oils with people with epilepsy. Each patient chooses an oil and over six to eight weeks has aromatherapy massage. The patients are taught, using post-hypnotic suggestion, to associate the smell with an intense feeling of relaxation. They carry the oil (either in a bottle or sprinkled on a handkerchief) wherever they go and when they feel a seizure coming on they sniff it.

The results have been remarkable. Of 50 patients treated in this way – all of whom had seizures that failed to respond to conventional treatment – 16 became free of seizures after a year (including three who came off medication completely) and in 17 the number of seizures was cut by half.

A trial was carried out in 1994 on 100 patients who had undergone cardiac surgery. They were randomly divided into four groups. One group received aromatherapy massage using essential oils, while another group was given massage with inactive oil. The third group talked with a nurse, and the fourth received no treatment. The physiological responses of each group were assessed by measuring heart and respiratory rates and blood pressure. Psychological responses were assessed through a questionnaire. The physiological effects of massage proved minor and not long lasting, while the psychological changes were clinically significant. A follow-up survey five days after treatment showed differences between the two groups that received massage which could be attributed to the use of aromatherapy oils. The results showed that aromatherapy had a significant beneficial effect in calming, relaxing and reducing anxiety of patients.

Can it do any harm?

Essential oils are extremely powerful substances. Bottles of essential oil are on unrestricted sale in the UK and need carry no danger warning. Some manufacturers do not include instructions for use. It *is* difficult to get detailed instructions on the side of a tiny bottle, but responsible manufacturers package their bottles in cartons with instructions wrapped round the bottle warning of any danger.

Essential oils pose several dangers, but these can be avoided provided they are used sensibly.

- Never drink an essential oil. Even in the small quantities in which they are sold – 5-15ml – pure essential oils can be lethal if drunk. If you drink them, you increase the risks inherent in the oil 10- or 20-fold. Essential oils are not medicine. Keep all essential oils well out of the reach of children.

- Never put neat oils on the skin.
- A few essential oils, such as cinnamon bark, can cause an allergic skin reaction. Essential oils are pure but this does not mean they cannot do damage. Always take care, particularly when applying oil to areas where the skin is damaged – burns or dermatitis, for example.
- Some oils are phototoxic. For instance, citrus oils in combination with sunlight can cause problems. If you have a massage with orange, lemon or bergamot oil and then lie in the sun for an hour you can burn, sometimes unevenly. This may leave permanent burnt patches on your skin. There have been a few instances, probably only a handful a year, where this has happened. Some essential oil companies seem unaware of this danger and offer no warnings.
- Beware of therapists who say they are going to give you a massage to 'get rid of toxins'. This is not the aim of aromatherapy. The body is full of toxins and is supposed to be.
- If you have high blood pressure, diabetes, epilepsy, a skin irritation or are taking homeopathic medicines, you should avoid certain oils – make sure you tell the aromatherapist if you fall into one of these categories.
- Pregnant women should always consult a qualified aromatherapist before using any essential oils.

How to choose a practitioner

Aromatherapy is unregulated: anyone can set him or herself up as an aromatherapist. But with the formation in 1991 of the Aromatherapy Organisations Council (AOC),* which in turn set up the Aromatherapy Trade Council* (see below), the practice of this therapy should be better controlled in the future.

The AOC represents 14 aromatherapy associations and over 80 colleges, which in turn represent 6,000 therapists – about 90 per cent of aromatherapists in the UK. When the AOC was founded, courses ranged from two days to two years: the minimum training stipulated is 180 hours in class. The AOC, which is developing national standards for aromatherapists, aims eventually to have one register.

What therapist you choose depends on what you want. If you just want a relaxing massage with good-smelling oils, someone who has undertaken a short course may be suitable. However, if you want anything more, it is important to make sure that the aromatherapist you choose is someone who has trained at an AOC-approved school.

Cost

Between £20 and £45 for an aromatherapy massage of 60-90 minutes is the norm. The length of treatment will depend on what you are trying to achieve. You may just want a relaxing massage, in which case one session would suffice.

For chronic conditions it is best to have a session once a week for several weeks, then once a fortnight, then once a month. Most people feel some benefit after a couple of sessions. Some people like to go for 'top-up' maintenance treatments, particularly if they have a chronic condition.

Buying essential oils

Essential oils are on sale in chemists, high street shops and supermarkets. Some outlets sell diluted essential oils. Not all manufacturers point out that their products are undiluted, and some 'aromatherapy oils' are synthetic.

Reputable companies sell pure essential oils and that is what consumers are used to. Oils vary enormously in price. Some are very expensive. If you find a brand of an essential oil considerably cheaper than the same oil in another brand, it may have been mixed with synthetic fragrance.

The Aromatherapy Trade Council (ATC) was set up in 1993. An independent self-regulating body representing 75 per cent of suppliers of essential oils, it aims to maintain high standards among its members and ensure quality in the products supplied to consumers. The ATC has drawn up definitions, used by trading standards authorities, of what constitutes an essential oil (for which the aromatic, volatile substance is extracted by distillation); an 'absolute' oil (which is obtained by solvent extraction); an aromatherapy oil (essential oil mixed with a carrier oil) and a perfume or perfume oil. Unfortunately there is still no definition of what an aromatherapy product is. There are toiletry and skin-care products on the market described as 'aromatherapy' products which may contain synthetic fragrance and just 2-3 per cent of essential oil. Others contain only essential oils.

ART THERAPIES

UNDER the wide umbrella of art therapies come music, dance and movement, drama and art. You do not have to be artistic, musical or graceful – or even have an ear for music or a love of dance – to gain benefit from these therapies. The art form is a means to an end; it will take you out of yourself and allow you to express emotions, such as anger and grief, which are hard to put into words.

The profession will shortly become state-registered and classified as a profession allied to medicine, which will make it illegal for unqualified practitioners to call themselves a therapist in any of these fields.

Art therapies can benefit anyone but they are used mainly with people who have mental or physical disabilities, emotional or learning difficulties, and those who are depressed or anxious or recovering from mental illness. These therapies give children and adults an opportunity to express the inexpressible, to articulate what cannot be said.

Central to all of them is the relationship between the practitioner and the patient or client, which should be one of mutual trust and understanding.

Theory, history and practice

Art therapy, a form of self-exploration through 'play', works by allowing people to express their feelings through painting, sculpting, modelling, collage and drawing. Clients are offered crayons, charcoal, clay and plasticine as well as paper, cardboard and old newspapers and can use the materials in any way they want to express their thoughts and feelings.

The therapist works with people, either separately or in groups, to explore the meaning of what they have created. Over a period of time the artwork can help the person learn all sorts of things about his life and get in touch with areas of his personality which may previously have been closed to him. Art therapists do not directly interpret the work.

The term 'art therapy' was first used in Britain in 1942, in connection with rehabilitating soldiers during the Second World War. Artists were keen to work with the sick and wounded and were employed under different titles in hospitals and clinics.

They began to be employed in the NHS during the 1950s and 1960s, but it was not until the 1970s that the development of postgraduate training in art therapy gave impetus to a movement for greater professional credibility.

The British Association of Art Therapists,* formed in 1964, pushed for art therapy to have a proper career structure within the NHS and in 1982, with the recognition by the Department of Health of the Diploma in Art Therapy, it achieved this goal.

Music therapy is well established in hospitals and now accepted virtually as a mainstream therapy. The ability to appreciate music, which remains unimpaired by handicap, illness or injury, may be the only thing that can alleviate pain brought on by physical or mental suffering. It has been proved to relieve the anxiety and fear that exacerbate pain.

Therapists work in hospitals, special schools, day centres and prisons; they can be employed by the NHS, the local education authority or social services department; and they also have private practices.

Music therapy can take place in a group or in one-to-one sessions. The therapist takes an active part by playing, singing and listening. Clients will not be taught how to play an instrument; rather, they are encouraged to use percussion and other musical instruments to create a musical language of their own.

A music therapist is usually part of a team, working alongside other practitioners, such as occupational therapists or physiotherapists, as well as doctors. For instance, music therapists work closely with speech therapists in a branch of music therapy called melodic intonation, which is used for people who have had strokes. Singing activates a different part of the brain from the speech centre, so music therapists teach stroke victims to sing and then try to switch the voice production technique to the speech centre.

While music therapists are holistic in their approach to their clients, they are also clinically directed and have specific aims and objectives. The terminology of music therapy is medical, as opposed to New Age, and compared with, say, sound healing music therapy is not an esoteric discipline.

Sound therapy or **sound healing** is different from music therapy. It involves the rhythmic use of sound to 'recharge' the brain with energy in a similar way to Gregorian chants, the Muslim call to prayer or Tibetan chanting. The therapy was introduced to the UK in the mid-1970s.

Sound healing is not for the sick and, although sick people may well benefit from the therapy, a reputable sound healer should not hold out the promise of a cure. The therapy is largely used by healthy people to 'widen their consciousness'.

People who want sound healing normally attend a day or weekend workshop, and will be taught how to chant from a repertoire of native American, Tibetan or Mongolian chants. Occasionally therapists use drums. Sound healers claim that chanting will make you still, centred, alert, empowered and relaxed. But the truth is that you do not have to go to a sound-healing workshop; you can achieve the same result by – say – regularly singing hymns in church.

Dance movement therapy, the newest of the art therapies to arrive in the UK, evolved from the theories of Rudolph Laban. Its aim is to enable people to express their feelings through movement. Classes start with loosening up. Then people are encouraged to use their bodies in a way that feels natural and comfortable to them. They may dance in a circle. Sometimes music is used to encourage movement; at other times the feet, hands and legs make the rhythm.

Dance movement is often used to treat people with psychiatric problems, from people who are alert but suffering from anxiety or depression right through to patients who are psychotic or severely disturbed. Mentally disturbed prisoners have also been treated by dance therapists.

Dance movement therapy has been shown to help with schizophrenia, anorexia and bulimia, and HIV and AIDS patients. It is also used with the deaf and blind, with children who have learning difficulties and with 'healthy' people who find that unchoreographed movement makes it easier for them to understand their feelings.

Therapists work in hospitals, day-care centres, prisons, schools and homes for the elderly. They sometimes work with individuals but usually hold group sessions.

Drama therapy is the use of theatrical techniques and methods in a clinical or educational context. Therapists work with the mentally and physically disabled, people with learning difficulties and people with eating disorders. They work with families, groups and individuals. Like other art therapists they work in hospitals, day-care centres, special schools, prisons and psychiatric hospitals.

Patients may be encouraged to act out a number of characters and explore different parts of their personalities, which are given expression through the text. The therapist uses different theatre genres – melodrama, Jacobean or ancient Greek, for example – to suit an individual or group.

What and whom they might be good for

For people who find verbal communication difficult, art therapies can be enormously beneficial. Music, for instance, can convey feelings without words. For someone whose difficulties are largely emotional it is a safe way to express repressed feelings. Music therapists maintain their therapy is particularly beneficial for children and adults with physical and learning disabilities.

Dance has been found to be good for depression and anxiety, the blind, people with physical and mental disabilities, people who are autistic and those who have learning or behavioural problems.

Art therapy is said to benefit people who are suffering from drug or alcohol addiction or eating disorders, and those who have difficulty in expressing their feelings. Therapists are now recognised and accepted on many NHS psychiatric wards, where they work with people with serious mental illness, including psychosis. Art therapy is helpful for a wide range of people with emotional difficulties, such as depression, anxiety and loss and bereavement.

Elderly people who have to cope with experiences that would shake most people at other times of their life, such as losing their home and moving into institutional care, find art therapy a good way of expressing their emotions.

How to choose a practitioner

All the art therapies have well-organised professional bodies, many of them established for over 20 years, which hold registers of qualified therapists. There are between 100 and 300 members in music, drama and dance and movement therapy and about 600 art therapists. These four art therapies are recognised by the Department of Health and have clear career structures, though some are longer-established than others. Qualified arts therapists can be recognised by the initials RATh (Registered Art Therapist), RMTh (Registered Music Therapist) or SRMTh (State Registered Music Therapist).

All the professional bodies require their practitioners to be graduates in the relevant subject – music, art, dance or drama – or an allied subject, such as psychology. Music therapists have to be trained musicians and are required to undergo five years of clinical training.

At the time of writing, proposals are being put to Parliament to extend the Professions Supplementary to Medicines Act 1960 to include art therapies (drama, music and art).

Cost

Music, art and drama therapy are available on the NHS. The sessions are usually attended once a week for an hour and the treatment may last for ten weeks or for years. Private sessions cost between £20 and £25. Sound healing is taught in workshops. A day costs £25–£50 and a weekend can cost anything from £80 upwards.

AYURVEDIC MEDICINE

ALTHOUGH ayurveda is little known outside Asia, and Asian communities elsewhere, it is considered by many to be, like traditional Chinese medicine, an effective holistic system of medicine. It is practised widely in Sri Lanka and India – in fact, the former even has a minister for ayurveda – and some doctors in parts of Asia switch effortlessly from conventional medicine to ayurveda, depending on what ailment is being treated. British colonisers closed down ayurvedic schools in Asia in the mid-nineteenth century, but the system of medicine survived.

The theory behind it

The word 'ayurveda' comes from two Sanskrit words – *ayus,* or 'life', and *veda,* meaning 'knowledge' or 'science': the science of life. Rather than alleviating or curing illness, ayurveda is designed to achieve a state of health through a blend of meditation, yoga, astrology, herbal medicine and dietary advice. It is the Indian version of aromatherapy, relaxation, herbal medicine, diet, and physical and spiritual exercise, all rolled into one.

Although ayurveda is distinct and separate from traditional Chinese medicine, the philosophy underlying it is much the same. Followers of both systems view the body as a microcosm of the universe, governed by energies, and believe that good health is achieved through a balance of these energies. The life force in ayurveda is called *ojas,* equivalent of the Chinese *qi.*

Ayurvedic medicine is highly complex and by no means easy to understand. According to early ayurvedic writings, each of us is composed of five basic elements – fire, water, earth, air and ether – which are converted by *agni*, the digestive fire, into three humours, or *tridoshas*, which influence our health and temperament. Air and ether yield *vata* (wind), fire and water produce the humour *pitta* (digestive juices), while earth and water combine to give *kapha* (phlegm). The character of an individual depends on his or her dominant humour. For instance, a person whose dominant humour is *vata* is likely to be creative, active, alert and restless. He or she tends to move and speak quickly, but also tire quickly. In physical terms, such a person is likely to be small-boned and underweight, and may suffer from arthritis and musculo-skeletal problems. If a *vata*-dominated person is 'balanced', he or she is likely to be vibrant, enthusiastic, imaginative and sensitive; when out of balance he or she will be restless, tired, constipated, anxious and underweight. When a person visits an ayurvedic practitioner (see below), the latter determines the patient's dominant humour and whether an imbalance of the humours is present. Food, drink, sensual gratification, light, fresh air and spiritual activities are used to produce the correct mix of humours upon which good health depends.

What it might be good for

It is claimed that ayurveda is good for treating a whole range of ailments: migraine; fatigue; chronic joint disorders, such as arthritis, rheumatism and gout; skin conditions, such as eczema, acne and psoriasis; indigestion, irritable bowel syndrome, stomach ulcers and digestive complaints; premenstrual syndrome, menopausal symptoms and irregular periods; and sexual problems such as impotence, premature ejaculation and infertility.

History

The earliest ayurvedic texts date from about 2500 BC, but ayurveda is believed to have originated in India in 5000 BC, which makes it the most ancient of all medicinal systems. It has been practised in the UK only since the mid-1970s, when many Asian immigrants arrived, and is slowly growing in popularity.

Treatment

On your first visit to an ayurvedic practitioner, you will be asked about your lifestyle, eating habits, relationships at work and family life. He or she will take your pulse the ayurvedic way and will examine your tongue, eyes and nails. He will also look at your build and features, and gauge your mood.

Treatment will take into account your constitution, the weather and season, mood and diet – anything that in the practitioner's view might affect your health. Detoxification is one of the main principles underlying ayurveda. Treatments used therefore include the application of warmth (*swedana*) or oil massages (*snehana*; see Massage) to improve the circulation, medicinal remedies and therapies such as yoga, meditation and dietary advice.

Medical products are prepared from plants using bark, root, fruit, leaf and sometimes seeds. Minerals, sea shells, animal substances and metals are also used. A health problem associated with excess phlegm, such as catarrh and water retention, for example, would be treated with warm, light, dry foods, fasting and the avoidance of cold drinks that would increase *kapha*. Herbal remedies might include hot spices such as cinnamon or cayenne, bitter ones such as turmeric, pungent tonics such as saffron and stimulating herbs such as myrrh, all of which are designed to clear excess water or phlegm. Taste is an important aspect of treatment in ayurveda. Bitter tastes can reduce *kapha*, so the diet recommended may favour these over sweet, salty or sour flavours.

You may be asked to visit the practitioner once a fortnight for the first few months, then once a month, depending on your health problem. The first treatment will last an hour; subsequent consultations will take about 45 minutes.

Does it work?

No scientific studies on the efficacy of ayurvedic medicine have been conducted in the West.

Can it do any harm?

Practitioners say that ayurvedic treatment has, by and large, no side-effects. However, researchers have reported that some traditional Asian remedies available in the UK are contaminated with heavy metals. Preparations used as tonics and aphrodisiacs appear to be particularly hazardous.

How to choose a practitioner

At the time of writing, there are fewer than 20 qualified ayurvedic practitioners in the UK. Each of them has undergone six years' training at a university in India or Sri Lanka. The Ayurvedic Medical Association UK★ holds a list of qualified practitioners. Most live and work in areas which have large Asian communities, such as London, Leicester, Birmingham and Bradford. Other practitioners of ayurveda have not undergone the full training, but have taken short courses.

Maharishi Mahesh Yogi, who founded the transcendental meditation movement (see Meditation), also runs centres for ayurvedic medicine, which he calls Maharishi Ayur-Veda.★

The Ayurvedic Company of Great Britain Ltd★ was set up by an international management consultancy, has four ayurvedic practitioners and runs a comprehensive database of herbal remedies. It treats the very wealthy, but will give treatment free to the elderly and unemployed.

Cost

About £30 for the first session, £20-£25 for subsequent sessions, plus herbal remedies, which cost about £10 a month. Maharishi Ayur-Veda costs £70 for a hour's consultation, with no treatment. Treatment involves three days' detoxification for £399, plus the cost of herbal remedies.

CHINESE HERBAL MEDICINE

CHINESE herbal medicine, which can successfully treat chronic diseases such as eczema, is one of the fastest-growing complementary therapies in the West. In the UK, Chinese herbal medicine has been practised ever since the Chinese community became established, but the herbs on which it relies became generally available only from the mid-1980s. Now some 260 registered Chinese herbalists practise around the UK, and between them they dispensed about 1 million prescriptions in 1995.

The theory behind it

Chinese herbal medicine, part of traditional Chinese medicine, has been practised for over 5,000 years. Practitioners believe that our health is determined by the state of our *qi* (pronounced 'chee') or vital energy and *xue* (blood), which must flow freely at the correct strength in the body for health (see Acupuncture for details). Any blockage in the pathway of channels along which the *qi* and *xue* flow, or imbalance in the components of *qi* (called *yin* and *yang*) results in illness. Chinese herbal medicine, like acupuncture, aims to restore the balance of energy in the body and nourish and support the constitution in a substantial way.

Herbs have one of five flavours (pungent, sour, sweet, bitter or salty), five *qi* attributes (hot, cold, warm, cool or neutral) and four 'directions' (ascending, floating, descending or sinking). The combination of these properties gives a herb a particular attribute or 'inclination'. In Chinese medicine it is the manipulation of these inclinations – following the principle of opposites – that brings about balance. Hence, a condition diagnosed as being 'hot' has to be 'cooled'; a 'cold' one 'warmed'; a 'deficient' one 'tonified'; an 'excessive' one 'purged'; a 'dry' one 'moistened'; and so on. For example, substances with 'ascending' or 'floating' inclinations, such as flowers and leaves, are light in weight and are believed to lift the *qi* and dispel diseases on the outside of the body. On the other hand, substances with 'descending' or 'sinking' inclinations, such as seeds and roots, have the effect of checking an overactive *qi* and are useful in dealing with nausea and dizziness.

What it might be good for

Chinese herbal medicine is claimed to be good for skin diseases, digestive complaints, menstrual problems including premenstrual syndrome, chronic bronchitis, allergic rhinitis, some kinds of asthma and conditions such as myalgic encephalomyelitis (ME). It is also used for children who suffer recurrent infections. In China, herbs are also used to treat hepatitis A and B.

History

Throughout history every culture has had its own form of herbal medicine. In China the *Huang-di Nei-jing (Inner Classic of the Yellow Emperor),* written almost 2,500 years ago and still regarded as the definitive work on traditional Chinese medicine, lists 12 herbal remedies. But the real father of Chinese herbal medicine is thought to be the Emperor Yen (Shen Nong, *c.* 1500 BC), who spent a good deal of time experimenting with herbs to see which ones worked. His words of wisdom, passed on orally from genera-tion to generation, were finally compiled into a *materia medica* in about AD 200, which listed 365 herbs and established the founda-tions of Chinese pharmacology.

The text was extended over the years, as further volumes appeared. Li Shi Zheng's *Beng Cao Gang Mu (General Catalogue of Herbs)* took him 40 years to complete. Although it was published in the sixteenth century, it remains an important text. The Western anatomical bible, *Gray's Anatomy,* used by many medical students, is a mere pamphlet compared with the *Beng Cao,* which consists of 52 volumes and 1,160 illustrations.

The first colleges of traditional Chinese medicine were set up in about AD 1200. In modern China, traditional Chinese medicine and Western medicine co-exist. Hospitals based on the former have departments specialising in the latter, and *vice versa*. Some doctors are qualified in and practise both systems of medicine.

Treatment

The first consultation with a Chinese herbalist, as with most complementary therapists, will be the longest, and could last up to an hour (see Acupuncture for details). The practitioner will ask you about your symptoms, medical and family history, lifestyle and diet, and will want to know whether your bowels move regularly, how you react to stress, heat and cold, and whether you are an anxious or tense person. A Chinese herbalist relies on his or her sense of sight, touch and smell for all the diagnostic information he or she needs, and will therefore look to see whether your eyes are bright and sparkling, whether your hair is shiny, how you behave – even how you smell and what your voice sounds like. Checking the tongue is routine in traditional Chinese medicine, as it is believed to be indicative of your state of health. Your pulse will be taken at both wrists.

Once your condition has been diagnosed, the practitioner will prescribe a mixture of herbs for you. You may get a sizeable bag of them (as whole herbs, roots or powders), with instructions for use. Depending on your condition, they may drain 'dampness' or clear 'heat'. They may 'regulate' the blood or expel 'cold'. They may 'tonify' the blood, *qi*, *yin* or *yang* or extinguish 'wind'.

You will probably be instructed to prepare a *tang*, a soup made from boiling and reboiling herbs. You will be told to drink a mug of this liquid a few times a day, usually before a meal, for a few days. The muddy brew is likely to taste unpleasant, but not unbearably so. The practitioner may prescribe some herbal pills as a tonic too.

It is unlikely that you will experience any side-effects, but if you do, stop taking the herbs immediately and contact the herbalist again at once.

Does it work?

Interest in Chinese herbal medicine is growing at a substantial rate, partly because it is very effective for certain types of diseases. This is particularly true of skin conditions which orthodox medicine cannot cure.

One of the few studies in the West to have tested the effectiveness of Chinese herbal medicine involved the well-known Dr Luo in Soho, London. Queues of people with skin diseases formed regularly outside her practice because she was reputed to cure seemingly intractable conditions. Her treatment was so successful that in 1992-3 it aroused the interest of researchers at the Royal Free Hospital in north London. They approached Dr Luo, who agreed to devise a limited number of standardised formulas for patients whose eczema and other skin conditions fulfilled certain precise criteria. A double-blind placebo-controlled trial was carried out on 37 children with severe and disabling atopic eczema. Each was given a mixture of ten Chinese herbs. Of them, 60 per cent showed improvement that researchers said was 'significant clinically'. The children who had been given the herbs showed greater improvements than the children who had been given the placebo. No side-effects were experienced at all. The same mixture was also used on adults with eczema, some of whom had suffered for years, and they too showed an improvement.

Can it do any harm?

Dangers can arise from two sources: untrained or poorly trained practitioners (see How to choose a practitioner, below) and adulterated, poor-quality or dangerous herbs.

Chinese herbs and herbal pills and preparations – which number about 3,500 – are imported into the UK, either directly from China or from Hong Kong and Taiwan. Fewer than ten importers and suppliers of Chinese herbal products are to be found in the UK, only two of which – East West Herbs and May Way Herbs – have quality controls in place. They import about 20-30 tonnes each per year and employ technically qualified people to make sure the herbs are authentic and not contaminated. They are the only members of the Chinese Herbal Suppliers Association, which was set up and is monitored by the Register of Chinese Herbal Medicine (RCHM,* see below). Smaller suppliers, many of which are just trading companies, rarely have any quality control.

Under Section 12 of the Medicines Act 1968, herbal medicines which are manufactured, sold or supplied by someone in a face-to-face transaction do not have to be licensed. A herbalist does not have to list the ingredients in any remedy he or she prescribes. The product's safety and efficacy are his personal responsibility.

The Medicines Control Agency (MCA)* is currently working with the British Herbal Medicine Association to formulate the correct protocol to ensure quality control and safety of all herbal products.

As with Western herbalists (see Herbal medicine), Chinese herbalists are under no obligation to clear what they prescribe with the MCA.

In addition to the lax licensing rules, there may be several problems with Chinese herbs:

- they may not be authentic. It is easy for suppliers to fake products exported to the West. Cheaper herbs may be substituted for expensive ones. In a survey conducted in 1995 on herbs sold in the UK, 10 per cent of the 300 herbs that were examined were of doubtful provenance

- the quality of the herbs may vary. Although the Chinese texts on herbal medicine lay down clear guidelines, the herbs used in the UK do not always meet them

- herbs, pills and tonics may be contaminated. Some Chinese remedies contain toxic substances which can be effective if used by highly qualified doctors. However, not many people in the West are qualified to use them. The herbs may contain, intentionally or unintentionally, potentially dangerous non-herbal substances, such as poisonous metals (lead, arsenic, mercury, cadmium and thallium), and/or conventional drugs (corticosteroids, paracetamol, non-steroidal anti-inflammatory agents, benzodiazepines). The RCHM does not approve of the use of toxic metals, or of remedies mixed with pharmaceutical drug products

- Chinese herbal remedies may contain products from animals, some of which may be endangered species. Ingredients could include rhino horn, tiger bone, bile from bears, musk from musk deer and scales from ant-eaters. The Chinese govern-ment has banned the sale of tiger bone and the British govern-ment has been active in prosecuting practitioners who stock such substances. More commonly used animal products are fossilised ox bones, deer antlers, dried cicada skins and buffalo horn. Herbal medicines may also contain shell from oysters, seahorses, turtles and cuttlefish. Again, the RCHM has a strict policy not to use any endangered species.

A five-year study carried out by the Medical Toxicology Unit at Guy's & St Thomas' Hospital Trust (see Herbal medicine for details) has identified a possible link between Chinese herbal med-icine (for skin disorders) and liver problems. Two patients have died as a result of developing liver failure. No single toxic herb has been identified in the cases investigated and the responses are thought to have been idiosyncratic – in other words, the patients had an adverse reaction to a substance that is normally tolerated well by most people. This idiosyncratic reaction can be identified early by monitoring liver function before and during treatment. The RCHM has advised practitioners of Chinese herbal medicine to monitor their patients' liver function and has introduced blood-testing procedures. It is also conducting a two-year research pro-gramme into the effects of herbs on the liver.

One of the most tragic incidents involving Chinese herbal medi-cine occurred in 1992 at a Belgian clinic. The people who ran it had changed the slimming formulation to include two Chinese herbs along with a mixture of pharmaceuticals and other herbs. One of the Chinese herbs they thought they had ordered was *Stephania tetranda*, or *han fang ji*; instead, they received from the suppliers a powder which contained *aristolochia fangchi*, or *guang fang ji*. The lat-ter contains aristolochic acid, which is known to be nephrotoxic. The result of this mix-up was that 70 young women who attended the clinic suffered kidney failure and required dialysis. Some were left with permanent kidney damage. The effect of the aristolochic acid may have been exacerbated by the other pharmaceutical/herbal ingredients in the concoction, for example, the potent diuretic acetazolamide. It was the misuse of Chinese herbs by people with no training in the discipline that led ultimately to the tragedy.

If you buy the herbs from a reputable company (East West Herbs or May Way Herbs), or if the practitioner is a member of the RCHM, you should have no problem. But be wary of herbal pills and tonics, unless they are prescribed for you by a qualified practitioner.

Safety tips

- Always ask for exact directions for use. You are entitled to correct and proper information about how the remedy should be taken and how often. In the case of herbal tea, you should also be told how to prepare it: how much of the herb you should use with what quantity of boiling water and how long it should be left to infuse.
- Store herbal remedies with care, as you would any other drug – in a cool, dry environment, well away from children. You can keep a ready-to-use herbal product in its own container, but store loose-leaf tea in a tightly closed tin. Do not store herbs in a plastic container.
- Do not keep herbal remedies for years. Some herbal remedies lose their healing properties if kept too long.
- If you feel ill or have diarrhoea when taking herbal remedies, stop taking them immediately, and tell the practitioner who dispensed the herbs and your GP. Reputable practitioners will tell you whether there will be any side-effects from the herbs you are taking and if you feel ill will check on your progress.
- If any medicinal product, whether licensed or not, has adverse side-effects, it should be reported to the Medicines Control Agency. In theory, if a particular herb is deemed to be unsafe it can be banned.

How to choose a practitioner

Chinese herbalists in the UK are not regulated as they are in the United States. Anyone can set up shop, order some herbs and start dispensing. According to the RCHM and a leading professor of pharmacognosy (the study of the effect of plant substances on the body), many people do just that.

Three sorts of Chinese herbalists practise in the UK – those who have had the full training, available only in China; those who have received a limited training in China and/or the UK, and those who have had little or no training. Many of the hundreds of highly trained herbalists in the UK practise in London's Soho and in Chinatowns in other cities. It is unlikely that such people are quacks or charlatans; most are well-qualified doctors. Indeed, such is the rigour of the training in China that they are possibly more highly qualified than their UK-trained counterparts.

However, there is no way of telling easily who is a good practitioner and who is not. Unless you have some knowledge of Chinese medicine, it is almost impossible to know whether a particular school or college of medicine in Beijing or Shanghai is reputable or not. The only way to be really sure of a practitioner's qualifications is to choose someone from the RCHM. Its members must have a minimum of five years' training, including three years in Western medicine. They adhere to a code of practice and ethics. However, only 260 out of the 650 current practitioners are on the register. Very few of the most highly trained herbalists belong to it.

The European Herbal Practitioners Association, a political union which represents 1,000 herbalists from both the West and the East, is working towards registration of herbal practitioners. It hopes to form an umbrella organisation for Chinese herbal medicine, ayurvedic medicine and European herbalism.

As mentioned earlier, the first session with a Chinese herbalist should take at least 45 minutes. Chinese herbal medicine is holistic, so be wary of anyone who has a specialised clinic, particularly one for skin problems, and who sees you for just ten minutes. It is crucial that the herbalist takes a full case history, otherwise you may be prescribed a potion that reacts with a condition that the practitioner failed to spot.

Cost

Between £20 and £30, plus the cost the pills and potions.

CHIROPRACTIC

IN A survey of *Which?* readers published in November 1995 (see Appendix), chiropractic was the second most popular complementary therapy used, and six out of ten readers who had used it said that their condition had improved. According to the British Chiropractic Association (BCA),* the largest body in the profession, some 300,000 consultations were carried out for back pain in Britain in 1993 and demand continues to rise.

Chiropractic is less well known than its sister therapy, osteopathy, but is following hard on its heels by becoming the second complementary therapy legally to regulate itself. The Chiropractors Act, passed in 1994, defines and protects the term 'chiropractor'.

Under the aegis of the Chiropractic Registration Steering Group, all chiropractic groups in the UK are participating in setting up a General Chiropractic Council, whose role is to regulate the profession and maintain high standards of training and competence among its members.

The theory behind it

The word 'chiropractic' comes from the Greek, *cheir*, meaning 'hands', and *praktikos*, meaning 'done by'. A chiropractor specialises in the diagnosis, treatment and prevention of mechanical disorders of the joints, using his hands to manipulate joints and muscles to improve function, relieve pain and increase mobility.

As in osteopathy, it is usually the spinal vertebrae which are manipulated. Practitioners believe abnormalities in the joints and muscles can be brought about through stress, poor posture, traumas and accident. While chiropractors focus on the spinal vertebrae, they also work on the muscles, ligaments, joints, bones and tendons. The thinking behind chiropractic is that minor spinal displacements can cause nerve irritation, which in turn leads to disturbances of the nervous system and eventually illness.

Practitioners maintain, therefore, that the adjustment of joints can also have a positive effect on the nervous system; it can even relieve conditions such as asthma and irritable bowel syndrome that are not musculo-skeletal.

There are two types of chiropractic – straightforward chiropractic and McTimoney/McTimoney-Corley chiropractic. The latter are particular methods of chiropractic adjustment that utilise extremely light and swift movements developed by John McTimoney and Hugh Corley.

What it might be good for

Chiropractic is claimed to be beneficial for people with neck, shoulder, back (particularly low back) and arm pains, tension headaches and migraine, joint problems, and sports injuries to the knee, ankle, hands and feet. Practitioners say it is also good for constipation, irritable bowel syndrome, postural problems associated with pregnancy and painful periods. Some also maintain that it can relieve asthma.

History

Chiropractic was developed by a Canadian osteopath, David Daniel Palmer. In 1895, he persuaded his office janitor, who had been deaf for 17 years, to let him manipulate his spine. The janitor told Palmer that he had lost his hearing after he had felt something 'go' when he bent down. Examining his back, Palmer found a misaligned vertebra. He adjusted this by manipulation – and the janitor recovered his hearing.

Palmer developed a therapeutic technique based on his discovery, and the name was coined by one of his patients. Palmer later set up the Palmer Infirmary and Chiropractic Institute in Iowa, USA. The profession has grown rapidly since then and now there are about 50,000 chiropractors in the USA treating about 20 million people a year.

The BCA was formed in 1925. Forty years later, in conjunction with European chiropractic associations, it opened the first recognised chiropractic college outside the US, the Anglo-European College of Chiropractic in Bournemouth.* In 1972, the McTimoney Chiropractic College was founded in Oxford by the chiropractor John McTimoney. The Oxford College of Chiropractic, which teaches the McTimoney-Corley form of chiropractic, was established in 1984.

In the UK there are now just under 1,000 chiropractors – 700 BCA members, 270 McTimoney practitioners and 50 McTimoney-Corley chiropractors.

Treatment

At the beginning of the first consultation, the chiropractor will take a detailed medical history, asking questions about your lifestyle, and observe your posture and walking. In order to show the muscles fully you will be expected to undress to your underwear, and a gown will be provided if you wish to use it. If you prefer not to undress, go to your appointment wearing leggings and a T-shirt and say so.

The chiropractor will probably ask you to slide your arms down your legs and raise your legs, to see what effect this has on the spine and how the joints work. He may also carry out X-rays and other standard medical tests, if necessary, so that other possible causes of your condition can be ruled out. If he feels you have an underlying disease that needs to be investigated, he will advise you to see your GP.

Much of the first session will be devoted to discussing your case, counselling you on your lifestyle and explaining how your spine works and why you are feeling pain. Treatment usually begins in earnest at the second session. You will lie on a treatment couch. (Note that chiropractors very often have special couches that can be raised to the vertical position to minimise any pain in getting on and off.)

Chiropractors use a variety of techniques. Many involve working on soft tissue (skin, muscles and connective tissue) to stretch and relax the muscles. They also use 'high-velocity thrusts' to adjust joints. This might be done two or three times in a session, down the back and to the neck.

The joint is pushed beyond its normal range of movement, without damaging it. As the thrust is executed, the joint surfaces give way, which usually makes an unnerving cracking sound. This is not the bones cracking, but is caused by gas bubbles in the synovial fluid within the joints bursting under pressure. The thrust is short and precise and it is not painful, or even uncomfortable, merely strange.

The McTimoney technique appears to the observer (and usually to the receiver) to be extremely light. The key to the success of the adjustments, however, is the speed, dexterity and accuracy with which they are delivered. McTimoney therapists specialise in one particular adjustment known as the 'toggle recoil', which effectively frees the joint and releases tension in surrounding muscles. As the manoeuvre happens very fast, patients feel almost nothing. Practitioners generally do not use very many high-velocity thrusts.

Chiropractors also treat musculo-skeletal problems in animals (horses, cats, dogs and farm animals) with the consent of the animal's veterinary surgeon.

After a chiropractic session, many people say they feel 'freed up'. Some feel revitalised, others a bit sore. Some people feel sleepy, others energised. Sometimes you can feel stiff and sore the next day, but generally the reaction passes in 12-24 hours.

Does it work?

Most people know someone suffering from back pain. According to the National Back Pain Association,* back pain alone resulted in 116 million lost working days in 1994-5 (it is the greatest cause of absenteeism). The cost to the NHS of soothing our aching backs is estimated at £480 million.

In 1995 researchers at the Medical Research Council produced the biggest endorsement of the effectiveness of chiropractic in a study comparing conventional hospital treatment with chiropractic for those suffering from low back pain. Some 741 men and women with the condition were assigned at random either to a chiropractor or to a hospital outpatient department. After three years, the improvement was 29 per cent greater in the group treated with chiropractic than in the hospital patients. Moreover, not only was chiropractic found to be more effective in easing pain, it also proved helpful in providing long-term relief.

Studies such as this back up chiropractors' claims that the technique can ease back pain. Increasing evidence shows it to be beneficial for other conditions, too.

Can it do any harm?

Chiropractic is remarkably safe. Although some 30 people have died as a result of spinal manipulation since records began according to international data and a number of serious complications have been reported, the incidence of problems is low bearing in mind the high number of people who visit chiropractors. Chiropractors assert that many of these deaths were caused by non-chiropractic therapists practising manipulation.

Compression of the arteries, which could lead to a stroke, can occur, particularly during manipulation of the neck area, but the risk of this happening is minute – one case per million. By contrast, according to the BCA, 15,000 cases of paralysis are recorded for each million people treated for neck pain with neurosurgery.

However, such incidences may be under-reported, simply because few people would make the connection between a stroke and spinal manipulation. In a recent study carried out among neurologists in California, 170 reported 55 strokes connected to upper spinal manipulation in just two years.

Chiropractic is not suitable for trapped nerves or people with osteoporosis. Any serious condition that requires surgery should not be touched by either a chiropractor or an osteopath. (For further information see Osteopathy.)

How to choose a practitioner

If you go to your GP with back pain you will usually be referred to a physiotherapist, who may have a long waiting list. But there is nothing to stop a doctor delegating treatment to a chiropractor: indeed, this is now being encouraged.

In April 1996, the Department of Health launched a pilot project among 28 GP fundholding practices across England to test the
possibility of buying the services of osteopaths and chiropractors.
In September 1996, the Royal College of General Practitioners
issued guidelines to GPs for the management of back pain. These
recommend manipulative treatment within the first six weeks for
patients who need help with pain relief or are failing to return to
normal activities.

Nevertheless, some GPs are reluctant to delegate treatment to
what they see as a complementary practitioner. According to
research carried out by the Anglo-European College of
Chiropractic, family doctors are not well informed about chiropractic treatment. Figures showed that two-thirds knew something
about manipulative therapy, 22 per cent were 'quite familiar with
it' and 16 per cent had 'only heard of it'.

Most people see chiropractors privately. If you do, check that the
practitioner belongs to the BCA, the Scottish Chiropractic
Association,* the McTimoney Chiropractic Association,* or the
British Association for Applied Chiropractic (McTimoney-
Corley).* Practitioners who belong to the BCA or the Scottish
Chiropractic Association will have undertaken a five-year full-time
BSc degree at the Anglo-European College of Chiropractic, or an
accredited chiropractic college outside the UK. Before they are
awarded their honorary DC (Doctor of Chiropractic) they have to
complete a postgraduate year in a BCA clinic. Most members of
the BCA regard their training as equivalent to that of mainstream
doctors, though to be fully registered as a doctor takes a minimum
of six years.

The McTimoney Chiropractic College course is at present for
four years part-time with extensive clinical commitments in the
third and fourth years. A fifth associate year must be completed
before the therapist is admitted as a full member of the
McTimoney Chiropractic Association. The Oxford College of
Chiropractic too has a four-year part-time course; it is affiliated to
the British Association for Applied Chiropractic (McTimoney-
Corley).

Under the terms of the Chiropractors Act 1994, all chiropractic
colleges in the UK have agreed that future educational standards
will meet those set down by the European Council on

Chiropractic Education in 1992, or the standards specified by the General Chiropractic Council. Both the McTimoney Chiropractic College and the Oxford College of Chiropractic are actively pursuing validation and accreditation of BSc degrees with the University of Wales and Oxford Brookes University respectively to satisfy this requirement.

Cost

According to the BCA, costs range from £17 to £40, with an average of £28 for the first consultation, and a little less for subsequent treatments.

COLONIC HYDROTHERAPY

SOME studies suggest that one in five people in the UK suffers from some sort of digestive disturbance which could be diagnosed as irritable bowel syndrome (IBS); others put the figure as high as one in three. At least 7 million British people regularly suffer from IBS symptoms – alternating diarrhoea, flatulence, bloating, constipation and wind – and it is twice as common in women as in men. Other bowel disorders include recurrent abdominal pain and performance anxiety diarrhoea – stage fright. The British have long regarded a regularly functioning bowel as synonymous with good health.

Although a 'normal' bowel movement does not necessarily mean once a day (it could range from three times a week to three times a day), in an effort to attain the once-a-day goal, one in five people in the UK regularly takes laxatives, usually on the quiet: a total of 20 million laxatives a year.

The theory behind it

Colonic hydrotherapy or *lavage*, also known as colonic irrigation, works on the principle that the 'unhealthy' colon is clogged up with impacted faecal matter, gases and mucus deposits which proliferate owing to the Western diet, which contains many refined food products. All this matter, therapists claim, becomes trapped in folds in the colon wall, leading to a build-up of toxins, inhibiting the natural movement of the gut and leading to constipation.

Flushing out the colon with what amounts to an expensive enema is said to remove 'harmful' bacteria and give 'good' bacteria, such as *lactobacilli*, a better chance to proliferate. The difference between an enema and colonic hydrotherapy is that in the former the tube is not inserted so far up the intestine and the water is retained in the bowel and expelled in the toilet. In the latter more fluid is pumped into the patient, through the whole length of the large intestine. The constant flow of water in and out washes the whole colon.

What it might be good for

Claims have been made that occasional but regular colonic hydrotherapy clears the skin, prevents headaches, improves circulation, helps in the reduction of weight, alleviates the symptoms of myalgic encephalomyelitis (ME) and lifts depression; the treatment is also said to relieve the symptoms of IBS, particularly if it is used in conjunction with herbal, dietary or homeopathic treatment, and to benefit those who have subsisted on a diet of junk food for many years.

History

Colonic hydrotherapy is not a new therapy. The Greek historian Herodotus noted in his writings that the ancient Egyptians purged themselves during every cycle of the moon, 'thinking this to maintain a state of health by use of emetics'. He wrote that in Egypt there was a physician – an 'enema-maker' – who had special knowledge of the lower gastrointestinal tract. In ancient China, purgation by enemas was used to relieve constipation, clear 'stagnation of food' and 'expel excessive internal fluid'.

References to purging by enemas occur throughout history and literature. The French poet Voltaire advised in the eighteenth century that 'one of the essential gifts one should look for in a wife is the ability to administer an enema daily and pleasantly' and, in what has to be one of the strangest foreign-policy strategies of the nineteenth century, Britain placed an embargo on the export of purgatives to Europe in Napoleonic times.

The 'benefits' of a regular enema were widely promoted in the UK early in the twentieth century. In London 'colon laundries' were set up to purge people of the contents of their colons, which were believed to be the source of many illnesses.

Treatment

On your first visit to a colonic hydrotherapist, the practitioner will take a full case history and explain the procedure. He or she will usually be trained in another complementary therapy, such as naturopathy, and will almost invariably give you advice on your diet and lifestyle.

You will be asked to lie on your side on a table, wearing a gown, and the therapist will gently insert a lubricated sterilised speculum a few centimetres into your anus. You then have to lie on your back with your knees bent up while water is gently pumped into the lower 1.5 metres of the intestine via a sterile tube, at a low pressure to avoid any risk of bowel perforation.

The tube in your anus is attached to two smaller tubes at the base (like an inverted Y). Through one of these tubes warm water is pumped into the large intestine and through the other waste matter is drained away. The therapist then lightly massages the stomach to stimulate the release of matter. The session takes about 30-45 minutes. At the end of it you are told to visit the lavatory to get rid of any remaining water and then given a *lactobacillus acidophilus* drink to 'restore' the gut flora.

People who have experienced colonic hydrotherapy say that the procedure is not uncomfortable. Most claim to feel light-headed and elated afterwards. Many have an initial course of six sessions, at weekly or fortnightly intervals, with a one-off 'spring-clean' every six months.

Does it work?

Colonic hydrotherapy can be beneficial for people who have intractable constipation which fails to respond to laxatives. However, most of those who have the treatment probably have normal bowel function. Many have colonic hydrotherapy to get rid of 'toxins'. However, the idea that the gut is full of toxins and bacteria which have to be flushed away to achieve good health is dismissed as nonsense by gastroenterologists: it is rather like saying the heart should be cleansed of blood. The colon is populated by a variety of bacteria, the main function of which is to break down fibre. Not only are these bacteria vital for digestion, but they appear to have a beneficial effect on the mucus lining of the guts. Flushing out waste matter removes the material on which the bacteria feed and can upset the delicate balance of the gut. Tampering with the bacterial tenants of our intestines is not recommended, and drinking a glass of *lactobacillus acidophilus* after flushing out the colon will make little or no difference.

Can it do any harm?

A carelessly executed colon clean-out may deprive the body of salt, water and potassium. Moreover, if the pressure of the water that is pumped into the bowel is too high, it can perforate the colon.

How to choose a practitioner

If you feel you must have colonic hydrotherapy, make sure that the therapist is a member of the Colonic International Association.* To remain a member of the organisation, the practitioner is required to attend a two-day seminar every year and have his or her premises inspected annually.

Cost

Between £30 and £60 per session, depending on where the practitioner is based.

COLOUR THERAPY

OF THE various forms of visual stimulation, colour is perhaps the most striking and powerful. Moods have long been associated with colour. Indeed, our language reflects this: we are 'green' with envy or jealousy, 'blue' when we are down and 'see red' when we are angry. A person who is deeply depressed is described as being in a 'black' mood, and when rage is all-consuming, one becomes 'white' or 'purple' with it. Moreover, interior designers and psychologists claim that the colour of a room has an effect on people sitting in the room: for instance, blue is considered to be soothing, green calming and yellow warming. Colour therapy involves the 'application' of colour in a number of ways.

The theory behind it

Rays at both the visible end of the light spectrum (the colours red, orange, yellow, green, blue, indigo and violet) and the invisible (infrared and ultraviolet) vibrate. Colour practitioners believe that each colour of the spectrum has its own unique vibration. Our bodies absorb these electromagnetic waves and emit them in the form of an aura.

The aura which supposedly envelops the body encompasses the mental, emotional and spiritual aspects of our being, all of which interact with the physical body, and is filled with constantly changing colours. These colours are determined by our mental, emotional and physical state, and also our spiritual awareness. According to colour therapists, if we become emotionally or mentally upset, a change in the auric colours results, which alters the vibrational frequency of the physical body. If this is not rectified, it will eventually manifest itself as a physical disease. Colour therapy sets out to alleviate the effects of disease by bombarding a part of the body or the whole body with a particular colour, which can actually change the molecular structure of the cells in the body and 'rebalance' it. Different conditions are believed to respond to different colours.

In addition to colour therapists, some psychologists specialising in colour will devise palates of colour to suit you, your home or your company. These colours are meant to make you or your workforce feel good. The psychologists claim that colour can be used in your home and choice of clothes to enhance your personality. Image consultants use hair, eye and skin colour as the key to determining which colours suit you; colour psychologists use them to reflect and reveal aspects of your personality. Particular personalities are attracted or suited to particular colours. The colour of femininity and unconditional love is, in keeping with the traditional Western view, pink. Purple is chosen by people who are spiritual, brown by intellectuals. The trick is to surround yourself with colours which 'vibrate' with your own personality and raise your spirits. Part of the reason why the countryside is so restful is because it is green, a colour which is easy for the eye to adjust to.

What it might be good for

Each colour is said to have a therapeutic use, some of which are specific (blue to treat high blood pressure or insomnia, for example, or to alleviate asthmatic symptoms, relieve stress and create a state of relaxation; yellow may be used for arthritis; orange to lift depression; green for anti-inflammatory diseases or for its beneficial effects in cancer cases; turquoise to strengthen the immune system). Other uses include violet, for hopelessness and lack of self-respect; and magenta for encouraging someone to give up undesirable habits.

Colour therapists do not claim to cure, but say they can improve a patient's health, and that if an illness is treated early enough it is possible to reverse the process of illness. They describe colour therapy as 'energy medicine'. Nevertheless, one leading colour therapist in the UK claims to have successfully treated autism, migraine, cancer, asthma and AIDS with healing lights, and asserts that the colour yellow helps sufferers of arthritis by 'dissolving the calcium deposits in the joints'. There is, however, no scientific evidence to back this up.

History

The walls of Egyptian and Greek healing temples were painted all over in colours which were significant in themselves and very deliberately chosen. In addition, the Egyptians used gems, thought to be pure concentrated colour, which they ground up and administered in powder form to sick people. In ancient China, people suffering from chickenpox were wrapped in red silk and put out in the sun. This seemed to prevent scarring. Tibetan teachings recognise the power of colour in meditation, as does Christianity. The brilliant colours filtering through the stained-glass windows of churches were believed not only to glorify the religious scenes, but to help the congregation pray.

The scientist and poet Goethe published *Die Farben Lehre* (*The Theory of Colour*) in 1810; a more recent writer on colour therapy was Dr Rudolf Steiner, founder of the Anthroposophical Society in Switzerland.

Treatment

The first session with a colour therapist takes about two hours. Gifted therapists claim to see the 'colour' in the aura that is said to envelop the body. Others may ask you to choose a colour from a range of cards or bottles filled with coloured liquid. The colour you choose is believed to reveal important traits of your personality.

The therapist will ask you about your health and whether you are taking any medication. Then he or she will decide what colours should be 'applied'. The main colour chosen is usually given with a complementary colour (for example, green with magenta), to enhance the former's power. Colour can be applied in a number of ways – through stained-glass filters either to the whole body or to a part of the body, or by laying crystals on the person. Other colour therapy tools include silk scarves and coloured water.

Does it work?

Although practitioners claim that colour therapy can help improve people's health, no scientific evidence exists to prove that it is beneficial. If someone is HIV-positive or has cancer it is highly unlikely that sitting in a green room will do much good, though it may help the person's mood. Colour therapy may offer hope where everything else has failed, but it offers only that, not a cure.

Can it do any harm?

Colour therapy cannot in itself be harmful, but practitioners are not clinically trained and may not be able to spot underlying disease. As with most complementary therapies it is important to see a doctor before seeing a therapist. People suffering from high blood pressure, epilepsy, heart disease and asthma should not be subjected to red light, while those suffering from depression should not be given blue light, as this can aggravate the condition.

How to choose a practitioner

About 600 colour therapists are to be found in the UK. Not all are qualified; colour therapy is unregulated and many unqualified practitioners can charge substantial sums of money for sitting you under a series of randomly changing lights.

The umbrella organisation for the therapy is the International Association for Colour Therapy,* founded by Theo Gimbel, who is generally credited with having introduced colour therapy to the UK, in the 1950s. He now heads the Hygeia College of Colour Therapy, which he established in 1971. This is the main college in the UK which trains people in colour therapy.

A person who wishes to get a basic certificate has to undertake a year's part-time course of academic and clinical work. On completing the course he or she is eligible to join the Hygeia Register of Colour Practitioners. For a diploma, a practitioner must submit a thesis of 25-35,000 words. The initials to look out for after a practitioner's name are H.Cert.C.Th (Hygeia Certificate of Colour Therapy), H.Dip.C.Th (Hygeia Diploma of Colour Therapy) and IACT (International Association for Colour Therapy).

After working for two years, a colour therapist can apply for membership of the Institute for Complementary Medicine* and to be placed on the British Register of Complementary Practitioners.

Cost

About £45 for the first session, and £25 for subsequent sessions, which last about an hour. Colour psychology can cost up to £80 for the first session, which may last up to three hours, and £40 for subsequent treatments.

CRYSTAL AND GEM HEALING

THE BELIEF that crystals, precious and semi-precious gems (diamonds, rubies, emeralds, etc. are all crystals) have healing properties has a long history. The beauty of emeralds, diamonds, sapphires and less valuable crystals goes some way to explain why they have been credited with mystical powers and why they appear so frequently in myths and legends. For example, emeralds were credited with the power to ward off epilepsy, cure dysentery and aid weak eyesight. Crystals and gems have long been used as potent symbols of power and authority: for example, the more encrusted with jewels a royal crown, the more powerful the monarch is seen to be.

The theory behind it

Crystal therapists believe that crystals contain 'ancient energy' which resonates with the energies of the body to bring about healing.

What it might be good for

Therapists maintain that crystals can alleviate spiritual, mental and physical ailments.

Treatment

You can either buy your own crystals or visit a therapist. If you choose to do the latter, on your first visit you will be asked about your lifestyle, diet and medical history, then to sit or lie on a couch or on the floor. You will not need to undress. The therapist may put crystals around you or on your body; the gems or crystals may be held either by you or by the practitioner; or the therapist may use a combination of these approaches. A session lasts between 40 and 90 minutes.

The skill of the practitioner is in choosing which crystal to use and applying it in the most effective way for the person being treated. The therapist channels the 'divine' healing energy to the person. Practitioners say the crystal acts as a focus; clients heal themselves and the crystal facilitates this.

Different stones are believed to be suitable for particular ailments. Quartz, for instance, is believed to be good for general healing while garnet is said to help depression.

Does it work?

Crystal therapists do not treat specific conditions. They take a holistic approach and claim that the therapy creates general well-being. Some people find that holding, wearing, being covered in or surrounded by crystals makes them feel better. But no scientific evidence suggests that crystals have healing properties.

Can it do any harm?

There is no harm in crystal therapy, so long as you consult a doctor if you feel unwell.

How to choose a practitioner

The Affiliation of Crystal Healing Organisations (ACHO)* was set up in 1988 to act as a representative body for crystal therapy. It represents eight crystal healing organisations. All the registered practitioners undergo a minimum of two years' part-time training, are insured and are obliged to adhere to a code of conduct.

Cost

Sessions cost between £10 and £30 depending on the area in which the therapist practises. Some therapists charge less for elderly and unemployed people. Crystals range in cost from 10p to tens of thousands of pounds. An attractive crystal to wear as a pendant will cost about £10.

FLOWER REMEDIES

THE USE of botanical products for medicinal purposes is ancient and universal. Although it is usually the green, leafy parts of plants that find their way into brews and concoctions, extracts from flowers are also thought to have a therapeutic effect.

The theory behind them

Flower remedies – of which the Bach Flower Remedies are the best-known – are 'extracted' from the flowers of wild plants, bushes and trees by soaking the flower heads in spring water in the sun for a few hours or by boiling the more woody plants. The resulting tincture, which is then preserved in brandy, is taken internally to lift the spirits, rather than to treat any underlying symptoms. The principle of the therapy is that our emotions have a strong effect on our physical condition, and lifting our moods with flower remedies should improve our health.

One of the attractions of these remedies is that a lay person can treat himself with them unlike, say, herbalism and homeopathy, which require trained practitioners to dispense the medicine.

What they might be good for

Flower remedies are said to help alleviate emotional and stress-related conditions. They are not used for specific physical problems: the aim is to 'balance' the emotions so that the body is free to heal itself.

Although the remedies are quite specific, some can be used for a variety of emotions. Chicory, for instance, is beneficial for tackling selfishness and possessiveness. For resentment, sulkiness and a tendency to blame others for everything, willow is recommended. Star of Bethlehem is good for shock and feelings of loss and is a vital ingredient in Rescue Remedy, a mixture of five remedies with which Dr Bach (see below) allegedly saved a fisherman's life in 1930. The purpose of the Rescue Remedy is to 'comfort, reassure and calm those who have received serious news, suffered a severe upset, or had a startling experience, consequently falling into a numbed, bemused state of mind'. Four drops is enough to revive a person, and it is claimed to work for animals and plants too.

History

Flower remedies are usually associated with Edward Bach (pronounced 'batch'), a Harley Street doctor, bacteriologist and later a homeopath. Born in 1887, he lived in London but spent much of his time in the country, walking in woods and fields. He discovered that when he became stressed, a walk would calm him; while out enjoying the fresh air, he found that he was attracted to particular flowers, which seemed to restore his inner peace.

He experimented by conducting tests on himself to evaluate the effects of dew gathered from flowers during his walks. He believed that the dew drew in the 'essence' of the flower and that flower essences could be used to lift people's moods and hence improve health. After abandoning his lucrative London practice in the 1930s, Dr Bach set about devising 12 remedies, based on the properties of flowers. To produce these, he soaked flower petals in spring water, dew being somewhat hard to come by in sufficient quantities. To these 12 he added a further 26, making 38 remedies in total. According to him, the 38 remedies used in combination cover all possible states of mind.

Dr Bach's work is continued by the Dr Edward Bach Centre,* now a thriving business. A large number of flower essences not included in his repertory are now marketed by other organisations. Some of these new essences were extracted by an American, Richard Katz, in the 1970s; since then, essences from all over the world, most notably Australia, California and the Himalayas, have been sold.

Treatment

Few complementary therapists use flower remedies alone; most of the people who use them in their work are qualified in another therapy, such as naturopathy, aromatherapy or reflexology, or are clinically qualified as nurses or doctors. However, as mentioned above, you do not need to visit a practitioner – you can buy flower remedies in many pharmacies. Before you treat yourself, consider your state of mind, your personality and what you wish to take the remedies for. Consult a practitioner if you are unsure of what remedy or combination of remedies to take. The practitioner will advise you on which combination is best for your emotional state.

You can also buy an empty 30ml treatment bottle and have the practitioner make you up a remedy for long-term use. To take flower remedies, dilute two drops of them in a glass of water and sip the drink as and when you need it; if there is no water handy the remedy can be taken neat on the tongue. You can take up to seven remedies at the same time, and can either buy the bottles separately or get the entire set of 38.

Do they work?

Scientific analyses of flower remedies show that there is nothing in them apart from alcohol and spring water. No clinical trials exist to show that they work. Despite this paucity of evidence, a surprising number of people, including medical practitioners, swear by flower remedies. This could be due to the placebo effect, or the brandy in which the tincture is preserved.

Can they do any harm?

Flower remedies are completely harmless and can be taken by anyone of any age or condition, even animals.

How to choose a practitioner

If you want to visit a practitioner, contact the Bach Centre, which keeps a list of 350 therapists who have completed its three-stage course successfully and have signed a code of ethics and practice. The Centre will also give free advice over the phone.

Cost

The remedies are fairly cheap: a 10ml bottle of one of the 38 flower remedies will cost about £3; a 10ml bottle of Rescue Remedy is about the same price, a cream costs slightly more. Advice from a practitioner registered with the Bach Centre will cost about £20.

HEALING

MOST people's image of a healer is that of a charismatic person who simply lays his or her hands on us and miraculously cures disease or other forms of impairment by means of some sort of spiritual energy, but this stereotype does not conform to reality. Plenty of anecdotal evidence exists about people who have seemingly been cured by the intervention of a healer. But can people really be cured by healers? Were their symptoms real or imaginary? Is successful healing yet another example of the placebo response at work? Or is there some external force at work for which scientists will never be able to find evidence?

The desire to be healed by means other than drugs and conventional treatment, and the belief that it works, are widespread. Healing is the most extensive therapeutic system outside mainstream medicine in the UK, where an estimated 20,000 healers of various sorts minister to hundreds of thousands of people.

The theory behind it

Healers believe that healing energy exists all around us: what they do is channel it to heal people. The energy helps repair the aura around a person which breaks or swells up if he or she is ill. According to some spiritual healers this energy comes from God; others maintain that it is 'cosmic' energy, which pulses through the universe. Some believe that the energy is a result of the interaction of the biological energies of the healer and the patient. The 'healing' of one individual by another without the use of medication or therapies can be done either from a distance or by the laying-on of hands, an ancient practice.

There are various sorts of healing.

- **Faith healing** This takes place in a religious context, usually during a church service, or in prayer groups.
- **Spiritual healing** The most common name in the UK for the laying-on of hands. Healing energy in this context is said to come from a divine source, but it does not require any faith on the part of the person who is being healed. A variation on this is 'absent' or 'distant' healing, whereby the healer, usually at a pre-arranged time, visualises the transfer of healing energy from himself to the patient, who does not have to be physically present.
- **Therapeutic touch** Similar to spiritual healing, except that the healer works just above the surface of the body. This therapy is widely used in the United States, mostly by nurses, and is based on the premise that a flow of energy exists between two people. The therapist places his hands a few centimetres above the patient and moves them over the entire energy field which is believed to surround the body. He returns to areas where he feels imbalances. Therapeutic touch is said to rebalance this energy field to bring about relaxation, pain relief and self-healing.
- *Reiki* A system of healing developed in Japan, it uses both the laying-on of hands and distant-healing techniques (see Massage).

What it might be good for

Healers claim that there are no conditions that cannot benefit from healing. Although conventional medicine should be the treatment of first choice for acute problems such as a broken leg or a burst appendix, healing can seemingly accelerate recovery and help a broken bone mend faster than it would otherwise. Some healers believe that they can put cancer into remission, although no reputable healer would say that to a patient: indeed, to do so would be illegal.

Healing is said to be beneficial for chronic conditions such as migraine and irritable bowel syndrome and for people who are physically and mentally disabled. Many people who use it regularly report feeling calmer, happier and more relaxed.

History

The roots of healing lie in religion, magic and shamanism. Most cultures embrace, or at one time have embraced, the concept of healing by a gifted person who is seen as the channel for energy from a divine source. There have always been healers, Jesus being the most obvious example in Christianity, and special places believed to possess healing powers, such as Lourdes and other shrines.

Healers flourished in the Church until the rise of Protestantism, which regarded healing (and still does) as a relic of Rome. Objections to healing come from both the medical establishment and certain Christian sects. Most churches have investigated spiritual healing and felt unable to endorse it, with the result that many spiritualists have broken away to form new churches in which they hold healing sessions.

Healing became organised in the UK with the founding of the National Federation of Spiritual Healers* in 1955 by Harry Edwards. The best-known of British spiritual healers, Edwards regarded himself as a medium for the healing work of Louis Pasteur and Joseph Lister. These 'guides' worked through him. Edwards held huge meetings at venues such as the Royal Albert Hall in London, where men and women who approached the platform were seemingly healed. The aims of the Federation were 'the promotion and encouragement of the study and practice of the art and science of . . . all forms of healing of body, mind or spirit by means of prayer, meditation, laying-on of hands, manipulation, etc., whether or not in the actual presence of the patient'.

These aims did not impress the British Medical Association, which in 1958 reported that it remained unconvinced that healing could cure anything that could not be cured by medical methods. It did, however, concede that 'through spirit healing, recoveries take place that cannot be explained by medical science'.

By 1963, the Federation had over 2,000 members. Now demand is growing for healing to be given under the supervision of doctors. Since December 1991 the Department of Health has allowed spiritual healers to practise in GP surgeries, provided the GP is clinically responsible for them. Between 200 and 300 healers work in hospitals. Healing is usually carried out at the request of the patient. A patient in any NHS hospital can request healing as long as the doctor treating him or her is told.

Treatment

Although healing is often linked with the words 'faith' and 'spiritual', and prayer in itself is therapeutic, most healing takes place in secular buildings, not in religious ones. Healers work in a variety of places: at home, healing centres or even doctors' surgeries.

At your first session of healing, which is likely to last an hour (subsequent sessions could be as short as 15 minutes), the healer will ask about your general health, your specific complaint and whether you have seen a doctor. If you have not seen a doctor, a good healer will recommend that you do – be wary of one who does not.

During healing you will be asked to sit upright (although some practitioners may ask you to lie down), relax and close your eyes. Because healers believe that energy comes through them, they place their hands either directly on you or 'pass' them over you, a few centimetres away from your body. They say that they sometimes feel this energy themselves as pins and needles.

You might find that the healer's hands are hot; indeed, many users report a tingly, warm sensation. Some have a direct feeling of energy moving through their body. Others say they feel 'spaced out' immediately afterwards; many healers allow you to stay and wind down after a healing session. Many people report feeling energised and invigorated the next day.

In absent or distant healing the healer focuses on the patient and 'transmits' his energy to that person to bring about healing.

It does not matter if you are a complete sceptic although, as with all forms of treatment, mainstream or otherwise, a rapport with the practitioner and a desire to get better may help. It is also possible that another healer may be able to help. Healers say they are not in the 'miracle cure' business and admit that it does not work for everyone.

Does it work?

No one really knows how healing – especially absent healing – works. The idea that someone can treat the physiology of a person who is miles away cannot currently be explained. Healers themselves do not know where the energy comes from or how it heals. But plenty of anecdotal evidence exists showing that it does, and certainly people do experience 'healing hands' as hot. However, like drug therapy, healing does not work for everybody. Moreover, some people relapse after a few weeks and little research has been done to follow up healing episodes.

Healers claim that the energy emitted from their bodies is shaped by their minds to boost the energy of the person receiving it. Studies show that if the healer goes through the motions of healing but is doing mental arithmetic at the time, the healing is not successful.

Most doctors regard healing as just an example of the placebo response at work, or self-hypnosis, but many remain open-minded. Some GPs refer patients to healers. The Doctor-Healer Network, loosely affiliated to the Confederation of Healing Organisations* (see How to choose a practitioner, below), has 70 members, 30 of whom are doctors.

Substantial research has been done into the effects of healing. An annotated bibliography entitled *Healing Research*, published by Dr Daniel Benor, contains details of 155 scientific studies. Of the studies, 64 per cent concluded that healing had beneficial results.

Research into the benefits of healing is being conducted in a large general practice in Devon. Since 1992 a healer has been visiting the surgery one morning a week and seeing an average of five patients for 45 minutes each. It was agreed that the healer would see only those patients who had chronic conditions which had been present for at least six months and who had not been helped by other treatments, either mainstream or complementary. They included people with arthritis, depression, stress-related conditions, headaches, abdominal pains, psoriasis, myalgic encephalomyelitis (ME) and repetitive strain injury.

After six months, the seven doctors in the practice decided to review the project. The patients were asked to assess their symptoms before and after healing and to evaluate any change they felt they had undergone. The doctors found that 70 per cent of their chronically ill patients had improved, a total of 72 per cent showed improvement in their symptoms, with 32 per cent of these showing substantial improvement.

The doctors are now repeating this experiment and comparing a group of patients who are having healing with a group of patients with similar conditions who are not. They admit that it is impossible to tell what the active ingredient in the package is – the placebo effect or some buzz of energy being transferred from the healer to the patient. However, they point out that that does not really matter; what does is that they are achieving improvements. The results are good, both for the patient and financially. Healing has proved to be cheaper than counselling. Patients return from the healer calmer and easier to treat because they have taken on responsibility for their health. Complementary medicine, according to these GPs, offers more in its method than it does in its treatment.

It may well be that many of those using healing (like most other complementary therapies) get relief from their symptoms simply because they have the full attention of the healer focused on them and supporting their desire to get better. If that is the case, they might get just as much relief from a priest or hospital chaplain as from a faith healer. Prayer, which is after all an example of absent healing, has been shown to be beneficial both to the people praying and the people they pray for. More than 200 studies have found that people with religious affiliation tend to live longer and have healthier and happier lives than those who have none. Scientists suggest that this may be because people with faith tend to lead healthier lives and are less stressed than their secular friends and colleagues.

Repeating words – perhaps in the form of a prayer or a *mantra* during meditation – while sitting still will calm you down and lower the levels of adrenaline and other stress hormones which affect heart rate and blood pressure.

Can it do any harm?

Healing cannot cause any harm by itself. Indeed, so good is the track record of healers that their professional indemnity insurance is extremely low. However, because healing may release 'suppressed symptoms', patients may feel worse before they feel better. As emphasised earlier, it is important to continue with your conventional medication while using healing: be wary, therefore, of healers who raise false hopes or ask you to stop taking your medicines. No one should expect miracles from healing, because no scientific basis exists for what it can achieve.

How to choose a practitioner

The Confederation of Healing Organisations (CHO) is a good starting point for those who wish to find a reliable healer. It is the biggest umbrella group for complementary practitioners in the UK, comprising 16 organisations and well over 8,000 members. The largest organisation within it is the National Federation of Spiritual Healers,* which alone has 7,000 members, and there are bodies representing Christian, Buddhist and secular healers.

If you are unsure which type of healing you should try, the CHO will advise you on which healing organisations to contact. These in turn will give you the name of a healer near you. The CHO has a strict code of ethics. Healers are forbidden to promise a miraculous cure. Any who do will be 'struck off'. Furthermore, a healer must ask the person seeking healing if he or she has seen a doctor, and must not make a diagnosis. If the person refuses to visit his or her GP, the healer must record that. All members of the CHO have professional indemnity and public liability insurance. The CHO forbids its members to use initials after their name, because this might appear to lend them an academic status which they do not have. However, members can say they belong to the CHO or the National Federation of Spiritual Healers.

Healing is a gift which can be developed with practice. Those on the CHO books are interviewed, have written references from satisfied patients, are put on probation for two years and are required to take vocational training, which is competence-based. National Vocational Qualifications will soon be available to healers.

If you are not going through the CHO, be very careful about choosing a healer. Anybody, gifted or not, can set him or herself up as a healer and charge money for 'healing sessions'. Be wary of charismatic evangelist healers, particularly if they have a mass following. Many have enriched themselves from the donations of people desperate for a cure. Many cases have been documented of people who have died as a result of abandoning conventional treatment following treatment by a healer.

Cost

A session with a healer can cost between nothing and £60; the average is £20-£25. Very often healers practise their skills in their spare time and therefore do not charge, although they would welcome some contribution to their expenses. Some healers refuse payment because they feel it would be an abuse of their powers of healing, which they regard as God-given. Ask beforehand what the fee is and avoid healers who charge excessively. A GP can refer you to a healer under the NHS, providing the funding comes from the practice budget. If you do not feel any benefits after three sessions, you should question whether it is worth continuing.

HERBAL MEDICINE

LONG dismissed by some people as rooted in the superstitions of the past, herbal medicine, or phytotherapy as it is called in continental Europe, is becoming increasingly popular and widespread. The number of herbalists – 1,500 in the UK at the time of writing – is growing fast. Herbal medicine is used most in the north of England and in the Midlands despite the fact that complementary medicine is used twice as much in the south-west of England as in the UK as a whole.

Many people, both practitioners and consumers, are fiercely loyal to herbal medicine. In 1994 the Medicines Control Agency told herbal medicine suppliers that by 1 January 1995 every herbal remedy would have to be licensed, which would have meant the closure of many suppliers' businesses. The move was dropped because of the unexpectedly high number of people writing to the government objecting to the plans.

According to a survey published in *Which?* in November 1995 (see Appendix), only 6 per cent of the 2,724 respondents who had tried complementary medicine had consulted a herbalist in the previous year. Of those who expressed an opinion on herbalism, 78 per cent said that they were satisfied with the treatment and 71 per cent that they would recommend it to their friends.

While some people might baulk at visiting a herbalist, it does not seem to prevent them from buying herbal remedies. An estimated 5 million people in the UK regularly do so. In 1995 the market was worth £28 million and sales of herbal medicine are rising fast, reflecting our willingness to experiment with complementary methods of dealing with sleeplessness, listlessness and general aches and pains. Nearly every week new herbal products are launched on to the market to banish water retention, headaches, nausea or stress. They are often cheaper than prescription products and, understandably, many people can see no point in paying high prescription charges for sleeping pills, tranquillisers and painkillers when there is a cheaper, 'natural' alternative. Moreover, 'herbalism' is a seductive word. It conjures up a time when our lives were simpler and less busy, less complicated and less mechanised. Herbal medicine is free of additives and preservatives, perceived by many to be safe, rightly or wrongly, and therefore different from and better than orthodox medicine.

The theory behind it

Herbal medicine is the use of plants or plant remedies in the treatment of disease. Until the late nineteenth century, all medicines were derived from plants. As bio-medicine progressed, scientists learned how to isolate the active ingredients from the plants and then synthesise them in laboratories. Many orthodox modern medicines are of course based on plant remedies. The best-known of these is aspirin, similar to a substance found in the bark of a willow tree.

However, some medicines have unwanted effects. Herbalists treat patients with the whole plant, which has other elements in it that prevent side-effects. Practitioners argue that the balance achieved in nature cannot be reproduced in a test-tube. The medicines are taken as herbal tinctures and teas, and the theory is that they build up the body so that it fights off an illness or condition and heals itself. Of the thousands of plants and herbs a practitioner can choose from, most use around 200.

What it might be good for

Herbal medicine can be used for almost anything but it is said to be particularly good for skin complaints such as eczema and psoriasis, menstrual disorders, stress-related conditions, digestive disorders such as irritable bowel syndrome and stomach ulcers, and joint problems such as arthritis. Herbalists also claim success with people with high blood pressure, respiratory infections, sore throats and colds.

History

Herbal medicine is one of the oldest forms of medicine in the world and every culture has its own tradition of herbalism. Both humans and animals are drawn to plants to cure their ailments. Any owner of a cat or dog will know that when it feels off-colour it eats grass.

In England, herbal medicine was established formally by an Act of Parliament during the reign of Henry VIII. It is the only country in Europe in which herbalists can practise freely. The best-known work on herbalism is Nicholas Culpeper's *English Physician and Complete Herbal,* published in 1653. Despite the fact that over the centuries herbalism was often criticised by the Catholic Church and fell out of favour as medicine became more scientific, interest in it was rekindled in the 1970s, encouraged by the World Health Organisation (WHO).

Treatment

As with many complementary therapies your first appointment with the therapist will be the longest, lasting roughly an hour. The herbalist will take a full medical history, asking you about your diet, work and family life, your mental and emotional state, whether you have any illnesses and whether you are taking any medication. Herbalists are trained in conventional medical diagnosis, so the physical examination is much the same as what a doctor might perform. He or she will check your pulse, take your blood pressure and perform any necessary examinations.

Herbalists generally prescribe tinctures, which are herbs in alcohol and water, or syrups, made by boiling the herb in water and adding sugar as a preservative. Occasionally they may administer the herbs in the form of teas, poultices or ointments. They usually give advice on lifestyle and diet too.

Subsequent sessions with a herbalist last between 45 minutes and an hour and you will usually be seen at fortnightly or three-weekly intervals. Herbalists say that it would take no more than two or three months to get a significant improvement in someone's condition. You are unlikely to feel ill afterwards, but some people may get a touch of nausea or diarrhoea. If you do, go back to the herbalist immediately. He or she will probably be able to identify which herb is causing you problems and will vary the prescription slightly so that you can carry on with the treatment.

Does it work?

A considerable number of herbs and plants have been found to be beneficial to health. Any benefits are, of course, dependent on the quality and amount of the herb taken.

Echinacea purpurea, a large daisy-like flower, is used to strengthen the body's defence mechanisms and has proved effective in clinical trials. A recent analysis of 26 trials concluded that echinacea helps to stimulate the immune system. Long before penicillin became available, doctors were using this native American remedy to treat meningitis, TB, typhoid and diphtheria.

Garlic has been used as a medicine for centuries. Herbalists claim that it is beneficial for a range of diseases including high blood pressure, arthritis and asthma. Over 1,000 research papers have been published on the benefits of garlic.

Ginger helps nausea and may give relief for colds and 'flu.

Ginkgo biloba, particularly popular in France and Germany, is extracted from the leaves of the maidenhair tree. Scientists have shown that it destroys harmful free radicals (compounds which invade stable molecules in cell walls causing damage), helps the action of neurotransmitters in the brain, improves blood flow and acts as an anticoagulant. It is also thought to be beneficial in cases of tinnitus (constant ringing in the ear).

Ginseng has been used as a health-giving herb for thousands of years by the Chinese. It contains many chemical substances, vitamins and oils. Recent studies suggest that it strengthens the immune system and may also boost brain function.

Hawthorn has been shown to be beneficial in the treatment of congestive heart failure.

Mistletoe is used to treat cancer. It is now produced and marketed as Iskador, but trials testing its efficacy have so far proved insufficient or contradictory.

Peppermint contains menthol, which relaxes the smooth muscle in the gut, and is used to treat irritable bowel syndrome.

St John's wort has been the subject of many randomised controlled trials which have showed it to be effective in the treatment of depression. One of the active ingredients in the plant is hypericin, which has chemical and pharmacological properties similar to antidepressants. In a study published in 1996, researchers from Germany and the USA looked at 23 clinical trials involving 1,757 outpatients with mild to moderately severe depressive disorders. In 15 trials they found that St John's wort proved more effective than the placebo treatment and that it was also effective as an antidepressant. But they point out that further research is needed to determine whether the herb is safer than other antidepressants for patients with particular types of depressive disorders and what side-effects it may cause, and to evaluate the relative efficacy of different preparations and doses.

Herbalists claim that other herbs are beneficial too. Aloe vera and camomile are said to be good for healing wounds, capsicum for pain, valerian for insomnia, and feverfew for migraine.

Although many people disapprove of herbalism (in many American states it is illegal), the drug companies are paying unprecedented attention to it. In the early 1980s none of the top 250 pharmaceutical companies had a research programme involving plants; now over half have introduced such programmes.

Can it do any harm?

Western herbalism is, in general, very safe. The quality control on Western herbs is tighter than that on Oriental herbs imported into the UK. However, that is not to say that herbalism cannot cause any problems. As with any form of treatment, it must be used sensibly and with proper guidance.

The Medicines Control Agency (MCA)* regulates medicinal products for human use in the UK. It classifies some herbal products as medicines; they are licensed and tested for safety. However, an estimated eight out of ten herbal products are unlicensed. Some imported and mail-order products, used as stimulants, aphrodisiacs and tranquillisers, slip through the net completely. Although they contain powerful herbs they are unlicensed and go through no quality control. Some pills and tablets used in Eastern medicine may be contaminated with pesticides, fertilisers and heavy metals, such as lead and mercury. Moreover, under Section 12 of the Medicines Act 1968, a herbalist who makes products and sells or supplies them to a patient does not require a licence to do so. The herbalist does not even have to supply a list of ingredients, and the safety and efficacy of the remedy are his or her personal responsibility. However, if the herbalist simply dispenses remedies made by someone else, the manufacturer will come under the purview of the Act.

Although many people assume that herbal products are safe because they are 'natural', they are mistaken. The Department of Health has identified some plants that carry a potential risk. These include pennyroyal and broom, which can cause miscarriage; bearberry and ragwort, which have been linked to liver damage; and feverfew, which may cause mouth ulcers. Broom also causes jaundice. In 1993, comfrey tablets and capsules were withdrawn from sale in the UK because they contain pyrrolizidine alkaloids, which have the potential to cause liver damage.

Another common misconception is that because herbal medicines are good for you, you can take a lot of them. However, as with conventional medication, this is simply not true, and an excessive intake could be toxic. Moreover, many people are under the illusion that herbal tranquillisers are not habit-forming, but you can become dependent on something if you believe it is calming you down and helping you sleep.

The Medical Toxicology Unit of Guy's & St Thomas' Hospital Trust published the results of a five-year project on traditional remedies and dietary supplements in 1996. The aim of the work was to investigate whether the use of such products was associated with adverse health effects. Of the 1,297 symptomatic cases identified by the project in 1991-5, a possible or probable link was indicated between product and symptoms in 640 cases, and a confirmed link was made in a further 12 cases.

Another source of concern about the use of herbal medicines is that little is known about the interaction between them and conventional medicines. A single plant can contain more than ten active ingredients – for instance, a hormone to make it flower, or a natural pesticide – and one active ingredient in one plant could react adversely with an active ingredient in another. Another possible phenomenon is 'synergism', whereby the combined effect of two active ingredients coming together is greater than merely double the effect of the individual ingredients.

Some plants are known to react badly with particular drugs. For instance, kelp (dried seaweed) could interfere with the activity of antithyroid drugs, and ginseng may react with the antidepressant phenelzine. Herbs which contain large amounts of vitamin K could interfere with anticoagulant (blood-thinning) drugs.

Safety tips

- Never buy herbs or herbal products abroad, particularly in Asia, Africa or South America.
- Never buy herbal products by mail order, particularly from abroad. You will have no guarantee that they are safe.
- Buy a herbal remedy only if the package states clearly which herbs it contains.
- Do not collect herbs in the wild unless you know what you are looking for. Telling a poisonous plant from a non-poisonous one is not easy.
- Do not use herbal remedies for serious illnesses. Over-the-counter remedies are not meant for serious disorders such as diabetes, epilepsy or high blood pressure, or cancer.
- Stop using a herbal remedy if you start experiencing side-effects.
- Do not exceed the stated dose. Herbs can have serious side-effects if taken in large doses.
- Do not take herbal remedies for prolonged periods. It is not known whether it is safe to take remedies over a number of years.
- If you are pregnant or are breast-feeding, in general do not use herbal remedies. If you do want to do so, ask your GP or a qualified medical herbalist first. Many herbal remedies should not be taken during pregnancy.

How to choose a practitioner

Anyone can set up as a herbalist and start dispensing medication with no training at all, so it is important that the practitioner you choose is a member of the National Institute of Medical Herbalists.* This is the leading professional body for European herbalism in the UK. All its members must adhere to a code of practice and ethics, and membership automatically includes professional indemnity. They generally have the initials MNIMH (Member of the National Institute of Medical Herbalists) after their names.

Membership is open to graduates of the School of Phytotherapy, East Sussex, and Middlesex University, north London. Both these institutions offer a four-year BSc degree course in herbal medicine, incorporating the mainstream medical sciences (anatomy, physiology, biochemistry, etc.), diagnostic skills, pharmacy and herbal *materia medica*, plus a minimum of 500 hours of clinical supervision. In addition, the School of Phytotherapy offers a course for GPs and two correspondence courses in herbal medicine that are 12 months and four years long.

No single umbrella organisation represents both Western and Oriental herbal medicine, but the European Herbal Practitioners Association (formerly known as the Herbal Practitioners Alliance), which has 1,000 herbalists, is campaigning for the formation of just such a body, which will encompass Chinese herbal medicine, ayurvedic medicine, *kampo* (Japanese) medicine and Western herbalism.

Cost

About £20-£30 for the first appointment, but with tinctures and syrups this may rise to £40. Subsequent appointments may cost £12-£15. You are unlikely to get herbal medicine on the NHS.

HOMEOPATHY

HOMEOPATHY is one of the most popular complementary therapies in the UK. Some 16 per cent of respondents to a *Which?* survey in 1995 (see Appendix) who had ever used complementary medicine had tried it, making it the third most-used therapy after osteopathy and chiropractic. Over the years it has had many royal adherents (HM the Queen is said never to travel far without her leather case of homeopathic remedies).

Homeopathy is unique in complementary medicine in having a Faculty of Homoeopathy* established by an Act of Parliament to train and register medical practitioners in homeopathy. There are five NHS homeopathic hospitals in the UK, in London, Glasgow, Liverpool, Bristol and Tunbridge Wells. The restructuring of the NHS and the formation of health trusts have put such establishments as the Royal London Homoeopathic Hospital (the second-smallest trust in the UK) on a much firmer footing. Its turnover rose by 25 per cent in 1995 over 1994. In 1994, 26,000 patients were treated at the hospital; by late 1996 that figure had risen to 30,000. Before the hospital became a trust, it was starved of funds from the district health authority because district managers felt there was not much call for complementary medicine; now it is paid for the number of patients it sees and the demand is considerable. Between 1988 and 1993 the demand at the Glasgow Homoeopathic Hospital increased by 40 per cent; the hospital deals, on average, with 220 referrals a month, nearly 90 per cent of them from GPs.

Even the natural scepticism – indeed, hostility – of parts of the medical profession is beginning to dwindle. The number of family doctors who want to take a course in homeopathy has doubled.

A study carried out by the University of Sheffield among 760 GPs found that acupuncture and homeopathy were the complementary therapies most commonly offered within practices and also the therapies for which NHS referrals are most commonly made.

The theory behind it

The word homeopathy is derived from the Greek *homoios,* meaning 'like', and *pathos,* meaning 'suffering'. The therapy is based on the principle 'let like be treated by like', an old medical tenet found as far back as the works of the Greek physician Hippocrates. The cure of the symptoms, and eventually the disease, is brought about by administering substances which produce symptoms similar to those which the person is experiencing. In other words, a substance that produces symptoms highly similar to the disease may also cure it.

Homeopathic remedies (tablets, granules, powder or liquid, which the patient takes by mouth, also creams and drops) are made from plant, mineral and animal substances. They are prepared by taking a solution of the concentrated ingredient (the 'mother tincture') and diluting it. At each stage of the dilution the preparation is shaken vigorously ('succussion'). Homeopaths believe that this succussion confers the therapeutic effect on the solution and that, ironically, the weaker the solution the more effective it is. However, these remedies are so dilute that it is arguable whether any of the original substance could be present in the medication in any physical form.

Two scales are used to express the strength of the remedies – the decimal and the centesimal. The gradation in the former is, as the name suggests, in tens, so a 1X dilution is a 1:10 dilution of the original mixture; a 2X dilution a 1:100 dilution. In the latter scale the steps go up in hundreds. A 1C dilution is therefore a 1:100 dilution and a 2C dilution a 1:10,000 dilution. For mild day-to-day complaints most homeopaths would recommend the 'sixth potency', i.e. a 6C dilution. More severe conditions would warrant a higher potency.

What it might be good for

Homeopathic remedies are thought to be good for hay fever, asthma, irritable bowel syndrome, eczema, migraine, premenstrual tension, stress-related problems and rheumatic conditions.

History

In the fourth century BC Hippocrates developed the proposition that treating a patient with something that mimics the illness might cure it, but it was a German doctor, Samuel Hahnemann, who established the principle for the modern world, in the late eighteenth century. Hahnemann trained in orthodox medicine, but became sickened by its brutality and lack of any sound philosophical and methodological basis. He abandoned his flourishing practice in Saxony and experimented with other ways of healing. In the process he discovered that crude doses of Peruvian bark (quinine) produced in himself all the symptoms of malaria, the very disease it was used to cure. As a result he published his *Law of Similars* in 1796.

Hahnemann believed that homeopathic treatment could kick-start the body into overcoming any health problems by itself, whereas traditional medicine works on the principle of nipping symptoms in the bud. As a trained scientist, Hahnemann subjected all the drugs that he used to trials on healthy people before administering them to the sick.

For instance, someone suffering from sickness, dizziness and indigestion might be prescribed the herb pulsatilla. In healthy people this produces virtually identical symptoms. These reactions were documented in homeopathic handbooks, compiled by healthy people who had taken doses of the substances. This process of recording evidence is known as 'proving'.

Hahnemann's remedies were all 'simples' – single, uncompounded substances, from animals, plants or minerals. He found that diluting the tincture did not weaken its potency; indeed, it seemed to increase it. Dilutions of one part in a billion still appeared to work, he insisted. Hahnemann called his method of diluting and succussion 'potentisation', a technique which allowed homeopaths to prescribe safely poisons such as arsenic, cocaine and morphine. He could not explain how the minute amount worked, but suggested that it might rally the body's defensive forces.

Hahnemann formulated three fundamental principles which are still the bedrock of homeopathy today:

- a substance that can be used to produce a set of symptoms in a healthy person may be used to treat a sick person who has the same symptoms
- potentising homeopathic medicine increases its curative powers while preventing unwanted side-effects
- homeopathy treats the whole person, not just the localised symptoms of the illness.

Homeopathy was introduced to the UK by Dr Frederick Quin, who after studying under Hahnemann returned to England in 1827 to become the first British homeopathic practitioner. Quin established the first homeopathic hospital, in Golden Square, Soho, London in 1850.

In the mid-nineteenth century homeopathy gained popularity, and during the cholera epidemic of 1854 the London Homoeopathic Hospital's lower death rate – 16 per cent compared to 60 per cent in general hospitals – did not go unnoticed.

Homeopathy spread throughout Europe, Latin America, the Indian subcontinent and the USA.

Treatment

A homeopathic remedy is specific to a particular person at a particular time. Some homeopaths maintain that every human being has a unique personal energy and a pattern of susceptibility to illness and other influences. This is manifested in behaviour, skin type, colouring, bodily structures and a host of other indicators. By matching remedies to specific individual symptoms, homeopaths claim to balance these energy patterns and restore health.

The homeopath takes into account your personality traits and habits, as well as the symptoms of your illness, and matches these to the remedies that he might stock – perhaps as many as 3,000 but usually no more than 40 or 50. Your initial consultation could take 1½ hours, during which you will be asked questions about your medical history, your diet, personal circumstances, work, moods, likes and dislikes, and sleeping patterns. Most conventionally trained doctors would not be particularly interested in whether you feel worse when the weather is colder, but the homeopath will want to know every little detail. Such a discussion might in itself make you feel better.

Using this information, the homeopath will choose the appropriate remedy. It might, like *lachesis* (snake venom) or *sepia* (cuttlefish ink), be derived from an animal; or, like *rhus tox* (poison ivy) or *aconite* (monkshood), from a plant; or, like *argent nit* (silver nitrate) or *nat mur* (sodium chloride), from a mineral.

You may be prescribed a single remedy ('classical homeopathy') or several remedies combined into one pill ('polypharmacy'), usually prescribed on an allopathic (i.e. conventional) diagnosis of a disease. Tablets are sucked or chewed on an empty stomach and for quick relief in an acute condition they need to be taken up to six times a day.

Some of those who try homeopathy feel an immediate improvement; others with a chronic condition are treated for months. Homeopaths subscribe to what they call the Rule of 12: that one month's treatment is needed for every year the person has had the illness. In other words, the rate of the response is proportional to the duration of the disease.

Some people find their symptoms initially get worse. This is called 'aggravation reaction' and, according to homeopaths, is a sign that the medicine is working.

Does it work?

Homeopathy seems to work, but no one knows how or why. The remedies are so dilute that under conventional chemical analysis they appear to be little more than water.

Moreover, the claim that the substance becomes more potent the more dilute it is is not explicable in terms of current science. According to conventional pharmacologists, homeopathy is nonsense because there is nothing of the original tincture.

Dr Peter Fisher, a consultant rheumatologist at St Bartholomew's Hospital, London, and a homeopath and research director at the Royal London Homoeopathic Hospital, uses the analogy of a computer disk when talking about homeopathic remedies. The disk may be imprinted with the complete works of Shakespeare, but in material and chemical terms it contains just vinyl and ferrous oxide, nothing more. Analysis would reveal that a homeopathic medicine contains water, ethanol (the medium in which it is diluted) and lactose (from which the pills are made) but also, according to Dr Fisher, 'information' stored in a physical form, which is not amenable to chemical analysis. This concept is now called 'information medicine'.

The body has powerful self-repair mechanisms, but they are sometimes 'scrambled'. This misinterpretation by the body is an important component in many chronic diseases, like rheumatoid arthritis, in which the body appears to be attacking itself, because the immune system has somehow become confused. Dr Fisher's view is that homeopathic medicine gives the body new and correct information, enabling it to heal itself.

Homeopathy is often criticised as imprecise, but actually requires great precision for it to work. Even if the right remedy is selected, it has to be administered in the right dosage. If homeopaths see no improvement they try different solutions until they achieve success. The fact that a result is not immediately obvious is, according to homeopaths, because the effects of suppressive drugs must be treated first, then, layer by layer, the underlying cause of the illness.

Homeopaths point to their success rate and the impressive body of scientific evidence to back their claims. In 1991, the *British Medical Journal* published a review of 107 controlled clinical trials of homeopathy and found that 77 per cent of them had positive results. The conditions covered included allergies, rheumatological diseases, respiratory infections, trauma, pain and psychological problems.

Critics argue that this is just the placebo response at work: if you believe something will do you good, it will. In 1986, however, a group of researchers from Glasgow compared the effects of a placebo and a homeopathic preparation of grass-seed pollen in 144 hay-fever sufferers. Neither the doctors nor the patients knew whether they had received a placebo or a homeopathic remedy. The people who had received the homeopathic remedy reported fewer symptoms, confirming the observation made by the doctors that homeopathic remedies have greater effect than placebos.

Moreover, trials on animals treated with homeopathic remedies are also producing evidence that homeopathy is more than the placebo response.

However, many scientists regard homeopathic remedies as little more than water. The seeming efficacy of the remedies may one day be explained by laws that have not yet been discovered.

Can it do any harm?

In itself, homeopathy cannot do any harm. It can be used during pregnancy and with the elderly and terminally ill. Homeopaths say the 'initial aggravation' – whereby you may get worse before getting better – may be distressing but is usually of short duration and never life-threatening. However, if you consult an unqualified homeopath about symptoms that should be seen by a doctor, you may be missing a tried-and-tested orthodox treatment.

How to choose a practitioner

There are two categories of homeopath:

- doctors with orthodox qualifications who are also trained in homeopathy: at present, about 300 medically qualified doctors are registered as homeopaths. Doctors who want to practise homeopathy undertake a six-month postgraduate course at the Faculty of Homoeopathy. Those who pass the examinations are entitled to register as members of the Faculty and put MFHom after their names. The British Homoeopathic Association* lists doctors who are registered with the Faculty of Homoeopathy. In addition, some GPs who are not homeopaths prescribe homeopathic remedies
- professional homeopaths, who are trained and who practise but who do not have medical qualifications. Make sure the therapist you choose is a member of the Society of Homoeopaths,* the professional body for homeopaths. RSHom after the name indicates that the practitioner is Registered with the Society of Homoeopaths, FSHom that he or she is a Fellow of the Society of Homoeopaths. Members will have undertaken a three-year full-time or four-year part-time course at a college approved by the Society.

There are also unqualified 'homeopaths' who are qualified neither in medicine nor in homeopathy. The field is currently unregulated and anyone can screw a brass plate to their front door and claim to be a homeopath.

The decision about whether to choose a professional or medically qualified homeopath is a personal one, but it may be wiser to choose the latter if you have a condition that needs to be monitored by a doctor. Homeopathy sometimes causes an initial worsening of the symptoms, which with a condition such as asthma or epilepsy could be serious.

DIY homeopathy

You do not have to go to a doctor or complementary practitioner to get homeopathic treatment. The remedies are available on the shelves of chemists and health shops and anyone can read a book on the subject and treat family and friends at home for simple, self-limiting complaints. According to a Mintel report, sales of homeopathic remedies increased by 18 per cent between 1992 and 1994 and were worth about £19 million in 1995.

Off-the-shelf homeopathic remedies come in two types: 'classical' or single remedy products, which are named after the remedy they contain; and 'indicated' or combined remedies, which are usually a combination of three or four single remedies that are suitable for treating a particular ailment.

There are two drawbacks to off-the-shelf remedies:

- they are not specifically tailored to you. Homeopaths spend much time finding precisely the right remedy to suit the patient: leafing through a flip chart in the chemist or health-food shop and picking a remedy can be a bit hit-and-miss
- consumers are not given enough information or advice to make an informed choice. A survey carried out in *Which? Way to Health* in October 1992 found that the standard of personal advice in pharmacies and health-food shops varied widely and that the leaflets and booklets given away or sold alongside the remedies often did not provide adequate detailed information. Indeed, the survey found that some leaflets recommended off-the-shelf remedies for conditions that were unsuitable for

home treatment, such as asthma, hay fever, skin complaints, ulcers and prolonged stomach pain or constipation.

Cost

The initial appointment with a homeopath costs from £20 to £90. Follow-up appointments are shorter and cheaper. If your GP is a fundholder, he or she can refer you to a homeopathic hospital under the NHS. If your GP is not a fundholder, the local health authority may have a contract with a homeopathic hospital. It is worth asking about an extra-contractual referral, known as an ECR. Homeopathic treatment is covered by most health insurance companies.

HYPNOTHERAPY

HYPNOTHERAPY did not fare very well in a survey of *Which?* readers carried out in 1995 (see Appendix). Among the 8,745 readers canvassed to monitor customer satisfaction with various complementary therapies, some 41 per cent who had had hypnotherapy were dissatisfied with the treatment, including 16 per cent who were 'not at all satisfied'.

The unpopularity of hypnotherapy could be attributed to the public perception of hypnosis as a technique that puts its subjects in a very vulnerable situation: the subject is perceived to have no control, to be under the power of someone else, and may perhaps even be persuaded to do something he or she would never dream of doing in a fully aware state.

These are misconceptions. A hypnotic state is *not* something that can be imposed by someone else. Hypnosis is akin to the trance-like state that we slip into every day: we can drive from A to B without remembering how we got there and carry out ritual tasks on auto-pilot, 'waking up' when we have completed them. We can be helped into that state by a hypnotist ('heterohypnosis') or taught to go into that state at will ourselves in a way that is intended to be therapeutic ('self-hypnosis'). Indeed, the training of people to use self-hypnosis is useful as it helps them understand that it is a state they achieve by themselves and that it has not been imposed upon them.

Hypnosis is about self-control. Undergoing hypnosis will not render you more liable to act out of character. No one can force you to be hypnotised; you can be hypnotised only with your consent. You do not have to be weak-willed or unduly compliant to enter into a hypnotic state. According to a study carried out by the World Health Organisation nine out of ten people can be success- fully hypnotised. It is usually those who are motivated and who are willing to make a change in their lives who are the most successful subjects. People who have a strong desire to be in control, particu- larly those who have disorders such as anorexia or obsessive com- pulsive disorder, are hard to hypnotise.

The theory behind it

Hypnosis is an altered state of consciousness brought about by deep relaxation. When you are hypnotised you are not uncon- scious; you remain fully aware of people around you, talking to you, and are totally relaxed, absorbed in the message you are hear- ing. You remain in control and no hypnotist or hypnotherapist can make you do something against your will.

Once you are in a relaxed state, the therapist will make sugges- tions aimed at helping you to change the way you experience or respond to something. No one knows quite how hypnosis works. One theory is that it calms and reassures the patient and this has a general beneficial effect. Another is that under hypnosis the left analytical side of the brain switches off, allowing the right, non- analytical, side of the brain to work.

What it might be good for

Hypnotherapy is said to be good for a variety of physical and psy- chological disorders. At the heart of hypnotherapy is relaxation; consequently it is used to relieve stress-related conditions, asthma, irritable bowel syndrome (IBS), rheumatism and arthritis (tension in muscles often causes a lot of pain) and angina. It is sometimes used for people suffering from multiple sclerosis, to help alleviate secondary symptoms such as stress and muscular pain.

Hypnotherapy is used for pain relief by dentists and surgeons, making everything from tooth extractions to giving birth less painful. Under hypnotic suggestion wounds are stitched, fractures set and burns dressed. Hypnotherapy can be used to make people less aware of pain and for that reason it can be used with those who are terminally ill to reduce pain and the suffering caused by it.

With children, who are very susceptible to hypnosis, hypnotherapy can be used to treat bedwetting and asthma and, again, for pain relief. Children can easily become engrossed in their own daydreams. Hypnotherapy, adapted for them with exciting, perhaps magical, imagery can be used to help them cope with dental treatment, or any painful or unpleasant hospital procedure. It can also be used to treat addiction and social problems such as stammering and blushing, phobias, panic attacks and obsessions.

History

The ancient Greeks used a phenomenon we might describe as hypnosis to cure anxiety and hysteria. The Druids used what they called the 'magic sleep' to cure warts. Magic, voodoo, shamanism, faith-healing and all kinds of ancient and primitive religious and medicinal practices have often incorporated hypnosis in some form or another.

In the late eighteenth century, a Viennese physician, Franz Mesmer, successfully treated a large number of people by putting them into deep trances. He called the technique 'mesmerism'. But his penchant for theatrical settings and ascribing the healing force first to electricity, then to 'animal magnetism', then to the power of the stars, soon alienated the medical community. *The Lancet* dismissed Mesmer and his followers as 'quacks and imposters'.

The real founder of modern hypnotherapy was a French country doctor, Ambroise Liebeault. According to J. Milne Branwell, who wrote the first major textbook on hypnotism, Liebeault would put his patients in a trance and then talk to them about 'the negation of all morbid symptoms . . . also the maintenance of the conditions upon which general health depends, i.e., sleep, digestion etc.'. Liebeault realised that it was because the trance made them receptive to what he said that their illnesses were healed. He used hypnotism to suggest that their ailments would resolve themselves – and the patients duly obliged. He explained to his patients that he possessed no extraordinary powers.

Hypnotism was brought over to the UK in the late nineteenth century by James Braid, a Manchester surgeon. He coined the term hypnotism (from the Greek *hypnos,* meaning 'sleep') and practised it frequently, even prior to surgery.

The medical establishment was unimpressed. Not until 1955 did a British Medical Association committee approve the use of hypnotherapy as a valid medical treatment for certain conditions. Some members of the medical establishment still distrust hypnosis. Since the 1970s, the new and expanding field of psychoneuroimmunology – the study of how the mind affects the immune system – has contributed much to the understanding of the link between mind and body.

In the UK, hypnosis is practised in the NHS by psychologists and doctors, but it is used more widely in the United States, Australia, Sweden and Japan.

Treatment

Do not expect dangling pocket watches or wagging fingers. All that is required is a rapport between the therapist and subject, a comfortable environment, free from distraction, and a willingness on the part of the subject to be hypnotised.

At the first session the hypnotherapist will take a full medical history, explain what hypnosis is and how it can be used in the patient's particular case. A session usually lasts 60–90 minutes and the average number of sessions needed to produce a result is between six and 12, usually once a week, depending on the condition which is being treated.

The therapist will encourage you to detach yourself from what is going on around you and to focus on imagery, thoughts and feelings. When you are relaxed, the therapist will make suggestions, or ask you to imagine certain situations. These suggestions might be accompanied by an image. If, for instance, you are suffering from eczema, you might be asked to imagine yourself bathing in a cool, crystal-clear, magic pool. If your skin is hot and itchy, you might be asked to imagine that you are rolling in cool, wet grass. Hypnotherapists sometimes plant a post-hypnotic suggestion that your particular symptom will get better, or every time you reach for a cigarette your desire to have one will evaporate or that you will have more confidence.

Does it work?

A 1992 report by the Royal College of Physicians on the use of complementary therapies in the treatment of allergies said that there was evidence that hypnotherapy could affect the temperature of the skin, and the sensitivity of the bronchi and gut; also, early studies of its effect on asthma were encouraging.

Hypnotic suggestion has been shown to affect the immune system by increasing and decreasing the skin temperature, speeding or slowing the heart rate and decreasing the secretions in the gut. Dr Peter Whorwell, a gastroenterologist at a hospital in Manchester, has been practising his 'gut-directed' hypnotherapy since 1984 and claims a 75-80 per cent success rate with his patients. In one study 15 people with severe IBS were given hypnotherapy. All had had a history of abdominal pain, bloating and erratic bowel habits for between two and 20 years (the average was nine years) and all had failed to respond to any other form of treatment.

A week before treatment, they were given a simple explanation of how the gut worked. The severity of their symptoms was recorded. In addition, another 'control' group was given the same time and attention as the first group, but no hypnosis. The controls were given a 'dummy' tablet which, they were told, would help their condition. The aim was to create a strong placebo effect, to make sure the patients receiving the hypnotherapy really were receiving something different. The hypnotherapy patients were given eight half-hour sessions over as many weeks, followed by two fortnightly sessions and one monthly session.

During the treatment, each patient kept a diary of his or her symptoms, recording daily the frequency and severity of abdominal pain, bowel habits, overall improvement of symptoms and well-being. Patients were judged to have improved only if their symptoms became mild or disappeared.

The results were remarkable. The control group showed a small improvement in all symptoms – except the important one, bowel movement. The patients who had undergone hypnotherapy all scored their bowel symptoms as 'mild'. The different scores between the two groups were statistically 'significant' – in other words, the change could not have been pure chance – after five weeks.

Eighteen months after the experiment first started, all those who had received hypnotherapy were in remission – free of their symptoms. Two had had a minor relapse, which was overcome by one additional session of hypnotherapy each. The overall success rate for the total group was 84 per cent, with classic cases (abdominal pain, bloating and abnormal bowel habit) achieving a 95 per cent success rate.

Hypnotherapy is particularly good for alleviating pain. In one study conducted over a five-year period, some 500 women giving birth for the first time were hypnotised during childbirth. The women all volunteered for the treatment and were given six sessions of hypnotherapy during their pregnancies. They were encouraged to learn and practise self-hypnosis techniques to use during labour when the therapist would not be present. The results showed that hypnotherapy shortened the first and second stages of labour in these women and reduced the need for painkillers. See Chapter 3 for further studies.

Can it do any harm?

Occasionally, hypnotherapy can be harmful. People with certain psychiatric disorders, such as schizophrenia, severe depression and personality disorders, should never undergo hypnosis.

Hypnosis may sometimes cause an 'abreaction', bringing back echoes of someone's past that may have been deeply disturbing. This could make the patient extremely anxious and frightened.

Hypnotherapists, particularly lay hypnotherapists, who delve too deeply should be avoided. A minority have become involved in recovering and reopening 'repressed' memories – events that may (or may not) have happened deep in the past and which are painful to recall.

Avoid stage hypnotism; you do not have to go up on stage to be hypnotised – even members of the audience can be hypnotised unawares.

If you have a chronic disorder, either physical or mental, go to a doctor. As with so many complementary therapies, if you diagnose yourself, visit a lay hypnotherapist and omit the safety-net of going to the GP, you could well be putting yourself at risk.

Hypnotherapy is little use if, for example, you are suffering from bowel cancer which you think is IBS.

How to choose a practitioner

Anyone can set himself up as a hypnotherapist. The UK has about 200 hypnotherapy organisations and between 4,000 and 5,000 hypnotherapists, many of whom are poorly trained.

The members of two organisations, the British Society of Medical and Dental Hypnosis* and the British Society of Experimental and Clinical Hypnosis*, are clinically trained – that is, they are doctors, dentists or psychologists with additional training in hypnotherapy. Together they have about 500 members, and they may merge.

At the moment no regulatory body exists for hypnotherapy. The only way to find out whether a hypnotherapist is trained properly is to ask him about his qualifications – but even that will probably not be very enlightening. Do not be fooled by a long line of initials after someone's name. One potential client plucked up courage and asked a hypnotherapist what the impressive-sounding LCHS after his name stood for and was told it was his motto – low cost, high success. Valid descriptions you may encounter are Reg. Hyp, meaning registered hypnotherapist; Acc Hyp, an accredited hypnotherapist; and N-SHAP, graduate of the National School of Hypnotherapy and Psychotherapy.*

Training for lay hypnotherapists can take anything from a weekend to six months part-time. Dentists, doctors and psychologists undertake training over several weekends throughout their careers. They are also expected to attend meetings, seminars and conferences regularly.

Many lay practitioners are highly experienced, competent hypnotists. Hypnosis is a skill that can be taught in a day and learned very easily. But it is wise to be treated by a clinically trained hypnotherapist, because the art of hypnotherapy is not merely inducing the state of hypnosis but knowing how to treat someone safely *after* they have been hypnotised.

You can be referred on the NHS to a doctor or psychologist trained as a hypnotherapist. Alternatively, the British Society of Medical and Dental Hypnosis or the British Society of

Experimental and Clinical Hypnosis can send you a list of clinical hypnotherapists in your area whom you can see privately.

Cost

Average costs are £30-£60 an hour. Beware of anyone who charges more than this. Treatment for relatively simple disorders and addictions such as migraine or smoking should need no more than six sessions. More complex problems, such as social phobias, may need more sessions.

IRIDOLOGY

MOST doctors would agree that our eyes are good general indicators of the state of our health. Many examine the eyes routinely. A milky ring surrounding the coloured part of the eye, the iris, is an indication of hardening of the arteries due to high cholesterol, or old age. Dullness usually points to poor health and brightness to the reverse. If the white of the eye has a tinge of yellow it is a sign of jaundice. An ophthalmologist, or eye specialist, will use a ophthalmoscope to look through the pupil of the eye for signs of diseases such as diabetes or a brain tumour.

However, while finding the eyes useful in diagnosis, few doctors would go as far as to agree that the body is, as iridologists claim, mapped out in the eyes or that close inspection of the iris would reveal the state of the tissues and organs of the patient.

The theory behind it

Iridology involves examining the iris for characteristic markings and colour which indicate the state of the individual's health and organs. It does not pinpoint specific diseases but practitioners maintain that they can identify physical weaknesses and underlying health problems which could lead to disease. The main message of iridology is that if you treat the underlying cause, the symptoms will go.

Each iris is divided into 12 radial sections, each section corresponding to an area of the body, such as lower abdomen, face or chest. Each segment is further sub-divided so that areas within one segment could cover the kidneys, adrenal glands, scrotum and so on. In addition, the map is divided into circular zones which indicate different tissues and body systems, such as arteries and blood, lymph, skin, etc. According to iridologists, the right iris records the organs on the right-hand side of the body and the left iris those of the left side of the body.

What it might be good for

Practitioners claim to be able to spot and alleviate general weaknesses in the body, such as hardening of the arteries, hyperacidity in the stomach and intestine, and weak kidneys. They say they can spot inflammation or the accumulation of lymphatic tissue, which might indicate underlying disease. If an iridologist feels that the disease could be serious, either physically or psychologically, he should, especially if he subscribes to a professional code of ethics, advise the patient to see a GP.

A good practitioner is well aware that iridology is a complementary therapy and is not a substitute for medical diagnosis, and patients should bear this in mind when consulting an iridologist.

History

Iridology was developed in the nineteenth century by a Hungarian doctor, Ignatz von Peczely (1826-1911). When he was a boy he tried to catch an owl, which put up a fight and plunged its claws into his forearm. The harder von Peczely tried to free his arm, the deeper the owl dug its claws in. The boy broke the owl's leg, and, so the story goes, at the precise moment he broke the bird's leg, he noticed a black streak appear in one of the owl's eyes.

He took the bird home, bandaged its leg and nursed it back to health. The following year the owl returned and von Peczely noticed that the black streak was now bordered by white lines.

When, in adulthood, he was consulted by a patient with a broken left leg, he remembered the incident with the owl and examined the patient's eye. He found a dark streak in the left iris and excitedly began examining the eyes of all his patients in the waiting room. In the years that followed he discovered a correlation between the markings in the eyes and the patients' diseases.

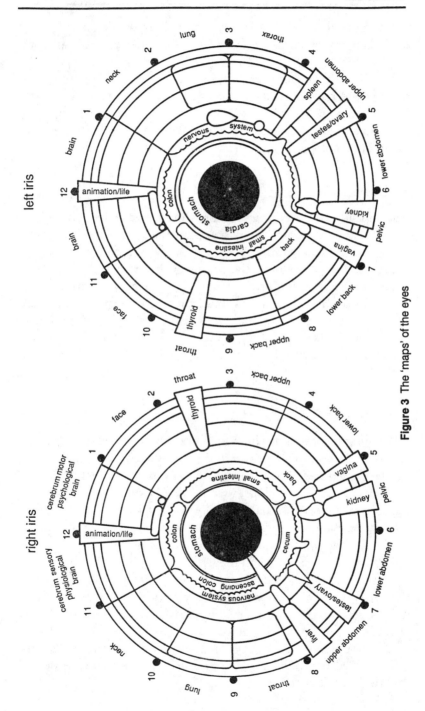

Figure 3 The 'maps' of the eyes

He drew up a 'map' of the eye, pinpointing which areas of the eye related to which organs, and published the result of his work in 1880.

In the 1950s an American physician, Dr Bernard Jensen, developed von Peczely's work, producing a more detailed map of each iris. These maps have been further refined and today practitioners claim that these charts enable them to detect past and future physical and psychological problems.

Treatment

Iridologists examine the eye using a torch and magnifying glass, then make notes of what they see. Some also use a special camera to film the eyes so that the patient can see what is going on.

Practitioners also look at the colour of the iris, which they claim should be clear and uniform, whether it is blue/grey or hazel/brown. A clear iris indicates healthy functioning of the major elimination channels in the body, such as the liver and lymph system. Once 'congestion' sets in and the function of the organ is affected, the colour in the iris will change in the area relating to the affected part of the body.

Does it work?

Examining the iris under high magnification is an everyday part of an ophthalmologist's work. Eye disorders such as glaucoma and retinal detachment can be diagnosed and many retinal problems are signs of other conditions, such as high blood pressure, narrowing of the arteries and diabetes. Operating on the iris is a routine procedure. But there is no scientific evidence to back up the claims made by iridologists, and ophthalmologists do not recognise iridology as having any place in medicine.

Some ophthalmologists report that they have examined patients who have been diagnosed incorrectly by iridologists, and whose irises were normal. The iris cannot develop new markings overnight; nor does it change colour, although it can do so under certain rare circumstances, such as a severe retinal problem. A condition called neurofibromatosis produces subtle abnormalities in the iris, but this is rare.

Few good studies of iridology have been carried out. A well-known one, by Dr Paul Knipschild, Professor of Epidemiology at the University of Limburg, Maastricht, showed that iridology is no better than chance in diagnosing gall bladder disease. The presence of an inflamed gall bladder, probably containing stones, is said by iridologists to be easily recognised by certain signs on the lower part of the iris of the right eye.

Dr Knipschild made colour slides of the right eye of 39 patients with this disease and 39 control subjects of the same age and sex who had healthy gall bladders. He distributed these slides to five leading iridologists, each of whom received a set of 78. Their diagnoses were no higher than might have been expected by chance and they were unable to distinguish the eyes of those with the disease from those of healthy subjects with any degree of success.

Can it do any harm?

Iridology should never be used in preference to conventional diagnostic techniques, such as medical check-ups, X-rays, barium meals, mammograms and blood tests. It is dangerous to rely on iridology for diagnosis. If you feel ill, see a doctor, not an iridologist.

How to choose a practitioner

Iridology is unregulated. About 300 qualified iridologists practise in the UK, but anyone can set him or herself up as an iridologist after a weekend course – or just a cursory reading of a book. Nevertheless, there are two organisations which hold practitioner registers and have their own code of conduct and ethics. The Guild of Naturopathic Iridologists,* which is affiliated to the Institute for Complementary Medicine, produces a register with around 70 names. All its members are iridologists who have qualified from what the Guild deems to be a good course, including its own run by the Holistic Health College, and they must have qualifications in at least one other therapy. Members are entitled to have R.Ir after their name.

One of the more prominent and most published iridologists, Adam Jackson, runs the International Association of Clinical Iridologists.* Practitioners on its register are graduates of its own college, the UK College of Iris Analysis, which Jackson runs. The six-month part-time courses are attended by complementary therapists rather than lay people. MCIrA after a practitioner's name indicates that he or she is a Member of the College of Iris Analysis.

Cost

£30-£50 for the first appointment, depending on where the practitioner is based; half as much for shorter follow-up sessions. Often one session is enough.

KINESIOLOGY

KINESIOLOGY is a system of natural health care which combines manual muscle-testing with the principles of traditional Chinese medicine. Like acupuncture, it works on the concept that disease results from blocked or imbalanced energy channels. Special techniques are used to unblock or balance them to restore the body to a state of health and harmony. The body has an innate ability to heal itself, according to the practitioners of kinesiology. By balancing all aspects of the person – structural, chemical and mental – kinesiology puts the body in the optimum state for self-healing. Enthusiasts say that this simple, non-invasive technique can reveal the causes of inexplicable aches and pains and general poor health, and correct them through a regime of gentle massage and touch.

The theory behind it

According to kinesiologists, certain muscles are linked by energy with acupuncture meridians, which are in turn linked with organs and glands. Through muscle-testing practitioners can evaluate the energy in the meridians and therefore in the organs. For example, the pectoral muscle is linked to the stomach meridian and the hamstrings to the large intestine meridian. If the pectoral muscle is tested and found to be weak, this could indicate poor energy flow to the stomach, which could impair health in the present and the future.

Kinesiologists use a range of treatments which, they claim, restore energy flow and muscle balance, including manipulation to improve nerve and blood supply; massage and touch to stimulate blood circulation and to balance emotions; and nutritional support and advice.

What it might be good for

Kinesiologists, unless qualified to do so, do not diagnose, nor do they claim to cure specific illnesses. However, they do maintain that their techniques can help with the many niggling emotional and physical problems that may lead to illness. They assert that kinesiology increases energy and vitality and can relieve aches and pains, tension, headaches, digestive problems, stress and emotional problems such as phobias, anxiety and depression.

History

The system was first devised in the 1960s by an American chiropractor, Dr George Goodheart. He was treating a man who complained that his shoulder blade kept 'popping out'. Examining the muscle that pushed the shoulder blade forward, Dr Goodheart was surprised to find some small, painful nodules at the point where the muscle appeared to be attached to the ribcage. When he pressed them they seemed to disappear and when he massaged them deeply the muscle itself became stronger.

He began experimenting. In his tests, he found that whenever a muscle became weak, the corresponding muscle on the opposite side of the body tended to tighten. However, when the weakness was corrected, the tightness was relieved.

He found that some muscles appeared to be weak because there was a sluggishness in the lymphatic system; when this system was stimulated by massaging specific reflex points, the muscles would strengthen. As he continued his research, Dr Goodheart found that muscles could also be weakened by a poor diet or from a blockage, and that correct diet and massage could correct these weaknesses.

Dr Goodheart developed a series of muscle tests based on the muscle/meridian connection. Instead of acupuncture needles, he used touch. He was happy to share and publish his work. Kinesiology has been practised in the UK since the mid-1970s.

Treatment

Compared with other complementary therapies, treatment sessions can be fairly long – an hour for the first and subsequent sessions. Much of the first session will be spent taking details of your medical history, diet, relationships, home and working life. Kinesiologists who are also osteopaths or chiropractors may take X-rays.

The therapist will then start testing the muscles. Unless he or she uses manipulation, such as osteopathy or chiropractic, you will not be asked to undress; testing can be done with the patient fully clothed. Most muscle tests are performed while you are lying down on a treatment couch, though a few will require you to stand.

The kinesiologist will move your arms and legs into particular positions and ask you to hold that position while he or she applies light pressure to the limb for a couple of seconds. From these tests, a kinesiologist can 'read' the body. A strong muscle will 'lock' or resist the pressure, a sign of health; a weak one will feel spongy and give way. Practitioners believe that restoring energy flow to the muscle/meridian will restore energy balance.

Kinesiology is often used to identify sensitivity to certain foods. The therapist may place a small piece of suspect food in your mouth or close to your jaw while testing the strength of a related muscle.

At the end of the first session, the kinesiologist will be able to give you a run-down of your main areas of imbalance and you may be advised to attend weekly for three or four sessions. You may also be advised to seek a medical diagnosis from your GP.

Does it work?

Many people say that they have gained benefit from kinesiology, but little or no scientific evidence exists to back up the claims of its practitioners. The claim that kinesiology can be used to pinpoint allergies, because the muscle strength will decrease if the patient holds a piece of food in his or her mouth to which he or she is allergic, was not confirmed by a double-blind experiment.

Allergens were first identified using kinesiology for 20 patients. Six patients were identified as having a 'positive' reaction to milk. When these were re-tested in a double-blind way, the results were no better than chance. Furthermore, when the experiment was repeated, different people were identified as having milk allergies. A number of other studies have shown that kinesiology is an ineffective form of diagnosis (see Bibliography).

Can it do any harm?

Kinesiology, if offered by a qualified practitioner, is harmless, and many people of all ages and states of health seem to have benefited from treatment. Be careful, however, if you have any recent scars or varicose veins, because these can be exacerbated by massage and pressure-point techniques (a trained therapist would know this anyway). Qualified kinesiologists are trained never to accept as a client someone whom they do not know how to treat.

How to choose a practitioner

Kinesiology is currently unregulated. There are about 600 kinesiologists in the UK and about 16 schools of kinesiology. The schools include polarity reflex analysis, applied kinesiology, biokinesiology, systematic kinesiology/balanced health, touch for health, and so on, but the principles are more or less the same.

The Kinesiology Federation* is an umbrella organisation which covers most of these schools. It has a membership of about 300 practising kinesiologists. The minimum requirements for membership are 150 hours of training and 200 hours of clinical experience within a period of two to three years. The Federation has codes of conduct and ethics, and a disciplinary procedure; its members (who have the initials KFRP after their names) must be insured. It is campaigning for a national curriculum for kinesiology.

The other main organisation is the Association of Systematic Kinesiology,* which has about 135 individual members. Training by this body takes 40 days, spread over two to three years.

Cost

Anything between £20 and £50 for a first visit and £15-£35 for subsequent visits. Most conditions can be treated in one to six sessions, each of which could, as mentioned above, last as long as an hour.

MASSAGE THERAPY

MASSAGE is still viewed in some quarters with suspicion. The British have a reputation for being reserved and do not give their bodies up lightly to strangers. The combination of touch and partial nakedness involved in massage has, for many, connotations of sexual intimacy. The proliferation of sleazy 'massage parlours', which have little to do with healing, has of course contributed to this national wariness.

This is unfortunate because massage is the root of all touch and bodywork therapies, which are recognised to be beneficial to health. Those who have experienced massage tend to become strong advocates of it. Massage is safe, soothing and non-invasive. For the healthy, it can be relaxing and invigorating; for the sick, intense, deep and intimate contact can relieve pain and, because it is so personal, alleviate loneliness where this is also part of the problem. Nine out of ten pain clinics in the UK have a massage practitioner.

The theory behind it

Massage (from the Greek, *massein*, meaning 'to knead') is a system of treatment by stroking, kneading or pressing the soft tissues of the body with the aim of achieving mental and physical relaxation.

A huge and increasing number of different types of massage are available in the UK, ranging from traditional Swedish techniques, through Thai massage to deep-tissue Indian *marma* massage. Some types concentrate on the muscles, others on the acupressure points. Some are soft and gentle, others vigorous, brisk and uncomfortable. Some focus on the whole body; others concentrate on the head, neck or shoulders. Some practitioners use just their hands; others use their elbows and knees. Sometimes the patient lies on a couch, sometimes on the floor.

Swedish or Western massage, based on body structure and muscles, tends to be used predominantly in sports centres and health clubs. Therapists use specific strokes to improve circulation, tone muscles, ease joints and smooth out knots in connective tissue. While some practitioners pay attention to the psychological and pleasure-giving aspects of massage, others concentrate on the more physical aspects such as improved blood flow.

Oriental massage works on the body points – usually either acupressure points or *marma* points (107 vital points, according to ayurvedic medicine, which correspond to organs or functions). The therapist may use his or her elbows and even manipulate the spine by massaging along it. Sometimes oils are used. The aim of the treatment is to release vitality and promote harmony in the mind and body. The main forms of Oriental massage found in the UK are Thai; Japanese or *reiki; tuina* (pronounced 'tweenah'); and *marma*.

Thai massage is practised on a mat on the floor (you should wear a tracksuit for the session). As in most Oriental therapies, the aim is to clear energy 'blockages' by a variety of techniques; the therapist uses the fingers, palms, elbows, knees and feet.

Japanese *reiki* (see Healing) is a form of touch therapy in which the therapist treats those parts of the body he or she senses are emitting weak energy, by laying his or her hands on or close to the site of the problem. This enables energy to start to flow through the therapist's hands to the patient.

Tuina is an intense and deep massage used in China alongside acupuncture or herbal medicine to 'balance' the energy flow. During a session of *tuina* you either sit on a chair or lie on a couch (fully clothed) depending on whether you are having your neck, arms, hands or back massaged. Instead of using the flat of the hands, a *tuina* therapist will push and twist into the flesh with the fingers, palms and knuckles. It is a vigorous but not uncomfortable procedure. *Tuina* is said to be beneficial for stress-related problems, neck, shoulder and back pain, sciatica, frozen shoulder and migraine.

Marma massage is a feature of Indian ayurvedic medicine (see Ayurvedic medicine). Stimulating the *marma* points is intended to bring about physical and mental well-being. A *marma* massage, for which you remain fully clothed, lasts for about half an hour. The practitioner will press parts of the back, neck, legs, arms and hands to unblock the *marmas* and thus improve the likelihood that you will stay balanced and healthy.

What it might be good for

Most people enjoy massage. Delivered sensitively, it will relieve illness in a number of ways. It is best for stress-related conditions, such as some kinds of headaches and insomnia. It can also be used to treat asthma, irritable bowel syndrome, constipation and digestive upsets, backache, sprains, strains and sciatica. In sport, massage is used to ease muscle tension.

It can also be beneficial for people who work on computers. Twisting your head to and from the screen, tapping the keyboard and moving the mouse can play havoc with the muscles. Regular neck, arm and hand massage can ward off repetitive strain injury. The lighter forms of massage, such as *reiki*, are particularly popular with the elderly.

History

The Greeks and Romans used massage to prepare their gladiators for battle, and both the Bible and the Koran refer to anointing the skin with oil. Massage was used in China as long ago as 3000 BC. Hippocrates prescribed it for his patients in 460 BC and urged colleagues to learn the art of massage. 'The physician must be experienced in many things,' he said, 'but most assuredly in rubbing.'

Middle Eastern and Asian cultures refined massage techniques, but in the Europe of the Middle Ages anything to do with physical and emotional pleasure was discouraged. In the nineteenth century a Swedish gymnast, Per Henrik Ling, developed a technique that became known as Swedish massage. Most European massage is based on this.

Massage was used in the First World War to rehabilitate injured soldiers. Archives show that nurses were trained in massage, while medical books published at the time reveal that it was used as a substitute for exercise to help victims of shell-shock, because it accelerates the blood flow to tissues, 'promotes the removal of waste products' and generally 'soothes or stimulates the nerves . . . and allays pain'. It was also beneficial in the treatment of fractures to alleviate pain. Until 1934, there was even a department of massage in St Thomas' Hospital, London. Massage methods formed the basis of physiotherapy.

After the Second World War, massage fell out of favour. It looked too primitive beside the new drugs and medical technology. Soon doctors had to all intents and purposes forgotten Hippocrates' advice about 'rubbing'. In the 1970s, massage again became popular. However, it developed a seedy reputation, which lingers – as a visit to any central London phone-box, where prostitutes often advertise their services by claiming to offer massage, will confirm. The words 'masseur' and 'masseuse' took on such lewd overtones that *bona fide* therapists now prefer to call themselves massage therapists or practitioners.

Today, massage is used by, for example, people who want to wind down at the end of the working week and those who want to give their body a treat and lift. You can go to a therapist, have one visit you at home, or even have a massage at your workplace.

Massage has once again caught the eye of the medical profession and now nurses and therapists in increasing numbers are employed in hospitals to treat the sick, the old and the terminally ill. It is available in pain clinics, hospices and residential homes for the elderly. Hippocrates would have been pleased that 'rubbing' is now back in favour.

Treatment

First, make sure you pick the right kind of massage for you: Swedish massage is best for relieving stress, while lower back ache or whiplash injury may require the deep tissue massage of the Oriental techniques. On the whole, Eastern massage tends to be more vigorous than Western massage. *Marma* massage, which clinics describe as 'brisk', can be positively uncomfortable.

As with most complementary therapies, the practitioner will ask you about your medical history, general state of health and perhaps your lifestyle. Mention any medication you might be on – and do not eat or drink immediately before a massage. It is important to be comfortable, so make sure you have emptied your bladder, and tell the practitioner if you feel cold/too warm during the treatment. Eastern massage therapists may look at your tongue and test nerve and muscle reflexes.

If you opt for a traditional (i.e. Swedish) massage, you can have either a full body massage or a neck and shoulder massage. For the full works, you will usually have to undress, but it is not compulsory. Most people leave their underpants on. If this embarrasses you, choose a therapist of the same gender as yourself. The therapist will use towels to cover areas that are not being worked on.

The therapist will usually treat the back first, followed by the neck and legs, using scented oils (or occasionally cream, body lotion or talcum powder) to help his hands move more smoothly. Then you turn over so that he can massage your front, shoulders, arms and hands. Massage begins and ends with slow, stroking movements to bring about a sense of calm and relaxation.

Most treatments take an hour (30 minutes for neck and shoulders only), after which you will be left alone for a few minutes to rest. You should feel warm and relaxed. You may feel giddy, light-headed or even sad – a massage can be an emotional experience.

You can have a massage whenever you feel you need one (usually between once a week and once a month). Some Eastern massage therapists recommend between two and six sessions to restore the body to peak condition.

Does it work?

Studies show that massage can help anxiety and depression and improve blood circulation. It is widely believed that massage helps relieve pain. This is partly because pain is often exacerbated by the tensing of muscles against pain: working to relax those muscles can bring relief. It may also be because massage is thought to release the body's natural painkillers, endorphins, which leads to relaxation.

However, according to an academically rigorous book published by Andrew Vickers at the Research Council for Complementary Medicine,* research on massage is disappointing, and good-quality clinical studies are few and far between. Vickers says that there is almost no good evidence that massage relieves pain; in his view 'the almost complete absence of reliable data' is 'disappointing given that massage is widely reported to be of short-term benefit for pain'.

That massage alleviates *anxiety* is better documented. A study carried out in 1995 by the Institute of Cancer Research's Centre for Cancer and Palliative Care Studies set out to evaluate the effects of an eight-week course of massage in 52 patients undergoing cancer treatment. The results suggest that massage has a significant effect on anxiety, assists relaxation and reduces physical and emotional symptoms. In another study, the results of which were published in 1992, 52 depressed people and children and adolescents suffering from adjustment disorders were given a 30-minute massage every day for five days. Compared with a control group who viewed relaxing videotapes, the massaged subjects were less depressed and anxious. Moreover, the nurses in charge of these patients rated them as being less anxious and said that the subjects' night-time sleep had increased over the period.

Massage is being used increasingly in cancer wards. Nurses at the Weston Park Hospital, Sheffield, currently use massage techniques on a number of patients – all of whom are having treatment for cancer – with considerable success and with the full approval of the consultant in charge.

Babies in incubators, sick children, heart and stroke patients, people with AIDS and patients in intensive care have also benefited from massage.

Can it do any harm?

Do not have a massage if you have varicose veins (although highly experienced therapists would know how to work around them) or inflammation of the veins (phlebitis), severe back pain (caused by, say, a trapped nerve, slipped discs or sciatica), blood clots (thrombosis), or a fever of any kind, or if you are in the first three months of pregnancy.

How to choose a practitioner

Massage is completely unregulated. One medical lawyer reports having dealt with several cases of people who had had back, neck and shoulder injuries as a result of massage. Incidents of this sort are extremely rare, but can happen if practitioners are unqualified.

About 200 training schools and colleges have been established in the UK. About 60 massage qualifications exist, and training can vary in length from a couple of weekends to a couple of years. There is nothing intrinsically wrong in a course lasting a few days that enables people to soothe and relax their subjects, or as an adjunct to beauty therapy. The danger is that sometimes people who have undertaken these short courses try to present themselves as able to treat a wide range of health problems.

The British Massage Therapy Council,★ established in 1992, should reduce some of the confusion. It is currently developing a register; meanwhile it has a list of 20 organisations and training schools and can supply names of local practitioners in most areas. Moves are afoot to establish a core curriculum and NVQ accreditation. At the moment, the Council recommends a minimum of nine months' part-time training.

The Massage Therapy Institute of Great Britain★ holds the names of 600 practitioners, many of whom trained at the Clare Maxwell-Hudson School, named after a leading figure in British massage.

Some practitioners may have qualifications from the International Therapy Examination Council (ITEC). It offers short basic courses in various body therapies, including massage. Five hundred colleges now offer courses leading to ITEC qualifications.

For serious ailments avoid massage that takes place in a 'health and beauty' context – and be extremely wary of advertisements in newsagents and *Yellow Pages*: it takes little imagination to work out what 'executive massage' or 'exclusive services' are.

Cost

Anything from £15 to £50, depending on the length of the session and the area. The average cost for an hour is £25.

MEDITATION

DESPITE the fact that thousands of people in the UK meditate daily, meditation still has a rather cranky image. It is one thing to have a massage or join a yoga class, quite another to sit cross-legged and intone a *mantra* twice a day. However, lowered blood pressure, deep and restful sleep, calmness, even heightened creativity and intelligence, and more, have been claimed for meditation.

The theory behind it

Meditation, practised regularly, aims to bring total relaxation, with all mental processes calming down, and inner peace achieved. During meditation the mind is released from any agitation, doing or striving, and is focused in the present, so that the meditator is troubled neither by memories from the past nor plans for the future.

Many types of meditation are available in the UK but the three principal ones are as follows.

- **Transcendental meditation (TM)*** is practised by many people to alleviate stress and is gaining acceptance in medical circles. Some 180,000 people in the UK practise TM. Each week 300-400 people learn the technique (but about 60 per cent of them give up doing it in the first year), which requires them to spend 20 minutes twice a day sitting comfortably with eyes closed and silently repeating a special word or *mantra*.
- **Buddhist meditation** usually does not use a *mantra*. In the basic Buddhist practices you develop awareness of breathing

and of positive feelings you have for people around you, even people you do not like. You seek to change states of mind that 'hinder' you from achieving peace and calm, such as hatred, doubt, desire, sloth and restlessness.

• *Mantra* **meditation** as taught by the School of Meditation* in London is a technique which allows the attention to rest on a simple sound to which you attach no attitude or emotions. It is essentially like TM.

What it might be good for

Meditation is effective in reducing anxiety and claims are made that it can alleviate the symptoms of disorders that may be stress-related, including migraine, insomnia, anxiety, depression, irritable bowel syndrome and premenstrual tension. It can reduce dependence on drugs and alcohol. Meditation can also lead to greater self-confidence and sense of self.

History

TM was developed in 1960 by the Maharishi Mahesh Yogi, guru to the Beatles, and was joyfully embraced by the hippies in the '70s. Buddhist meditation has been practised for over 2,500 years in Asia in both monastic and secular settings. In recent years, it has flourished in the West. The Friends of the Western Buddhist Order (FWBO),* an organisation founded in the UK in 1967, teaches two types of meditation: the *anapana-sati* or 'awareness of in-and-out breathing' and *metta-bhavana* or 'development of loving kindness'. The School of Meditation in London was set up in 1961 and has taught over 10,000 people since then. It runs courses in *mantra* meditation.

Practice

It can be difficult for a beginner to still the mind, so a teacher and the discipline of being in a group can be enormously helpful. But you can try meditation for yourself before investing time and money on a course.

Find somewhere quiet and sit comfortably. You do not have to sit cross-legged or in the lotus position: you could sit with your feet under your buttocks or astride some cushions or in a straight-backed chair. Whichever way you choose to sit, you need to have a straight back and to be able to sit for 20 minutes without the distraction of cramps and aches.

Your shoulders should be relaxed. Rest your hands on your lap or your thighs, so that the shoulders are loose. Now breathe deeply, filling your lungs and concentrating on the breath flowing in through your nose. Hold for a few seconds when your lungs are full, then slowly exhale. Repeat this ten times.

In some forms of meditation your teacher will give you a special word, or *mantra*. You can choose your own, such as 'one'; the name of a religious figure if you are committed to a religion; or a common *mantra* such as 'Om'.

Other techniques encourage 'mindful' meditation in which you focus on your breathing, or on a candle flame, crystal or icon. They all have the same purpose: to focus the mind. The philosophy behind meditation is that the mind is left free and moves towards a greater feeling of happiness or fulfilment.

Does it work?

It is claimed by some practitioners that during meditation people achieve a deep level of rest. This deep rest leads to the production of alpha brainwaves and changes in muscle tone and skin resistance.

A person may experience some of these variations, particularly an improvement in sleeping and a reduction in both anxiety and cravings if he or she is a smoker or heavy drinker, in the first few days after starting meditation. The benefits of meditation are, however, cumulative; the more you do it, the greater they are. There is some evidence that it may boost the neurotransmitter serotonin, in the same way as an antidepressant drug but without the side-effects.

Most of the studies attesting to the benefits of meditation relate to TM. This is not necessarily because TM is better than other forms of meditation but because the TM organisation has the money to conduct major scientific trials. Each European country now has its own group of doctors campaigning for the acceptance of TM – the UK has the British Association for the Medical Application of Transcendental Meditation with a membership of 700 GPs and hospital doctors, and in the Netherlands at least one insurance company is offering meditators a reduction of 20 per cent in health premiums.

Some 500 scientific studies on TM have been published since the mid-1970s in universities in 27 countries, all testifying to the efficacy of this form of meditation in dealing with anxiety, mild depression, insomnia, tension headaches, migraine, high blood pressure, irritable bowel syndrome, post-natal depression and a number of stress-related conditions.

However, TM does have its critics, who point out that most of the research is carried out by scientists who belong to the Maharishi Foundation, which is connected to the TM organisation, and that many studies are either published in journals which do not require a rigorous peer review or reviewed by other people in the TM organisation, thus lacking any objective viewpoint.

Scientific studies by non-TM people show very different conclusions. TM *does* reduce stress and *is* relaxing, but no more than sitting down and either reading a book or just doing nothing. Moreover, no evidence exists that TM is better for you than any other form of meditation. In any case, meditation is less effective in lowering blood pressure than is exercise.

The Buddhists are altogether more self-effacing and regard research to 'prove' the benefits of meditation as distasteful and little more than a sales package. The FWBO point to the positive experiences of the many people who attend their classes as proof of the effectiveness of meditation.

In the United States, a project using Buddhist meditation to control stress has been running successfully since the mid-1980s. The Stress Reduction and Relaxation Program, run by Jon Kabat-Zinn at the University of Massachussetts Medical Center, comprises an eight-week course based on Buddhist or 'mindfulness' meditation. Many of the people who come to the clinic have not seen any improvement in their physical condition despite years of medical treatment. At the end of eight weeks, the participants leave with fewer or less severe physical symptoms and greater self-confidence, patience and self-acceptance.

When the School of Meditation was founded, a research group carried out tests on meditators and found that meditation brought about a slower heart beat, decrease in basal metabolic rate and an increase in alpha brain rhythm. However, these tests were discontinued and the results were never published. The School lays stress on the effects of meditation on the subtler mental and emotional levels and less on the physical.

Can it do any harm?

Effective meditation brings about mental and emotional calm. However, if you meditate without the support of a trained and experienced teacher, worries and fears may surface that provoke more stress and even do harm. Those who are most vulnerable are people who are not facing up to what is happening in their lives. Those who meditate regularly admit that although painful memories may surface, meditation itself equips one with enough emotional and mental strength to deal with them.

How to choose a teacher

TM is taught in 50 centres across the UK. Go to an introductory lecture before deciding to sign up for sessions that will cost money. If you decide that TM is for you, you will probably attend four sessions on consecutive days and a further session three months later.

Buddhist meditation is taught by teachers in Buddhist centres across the UK. The FWBO runs 23 permanent centres in Scotland and England (6 in London, and 17 elsewhere). Other Buddhist organisations run centres too.

The School of Meditation in London holds introductory meetings or private interviews. Instruction in meditation is given at a later date, on an individual basis, in a session lasting 90 minutes.

Cost

Some fundholding GPs prescribe TM under the NHS, but this is rare. A course of TM (see above) normally costs £490 (£390 for students). A six-week course in Buddhist meditation, consisting of

2½ hours of tuition a week, costs £60 (£40 for unwaged people). For a week's meditation retreat you would pay £350 (£250 if unwaged). The School of Meditation requests a one-off donation of one week's income for the teaching of the technique and all subsequent guidance. Students, the unwaged and OAPs are asked to give £50.

METAMORPHIC TECHNIQUE

THIS is one of the hardest complementary therapies to explain and one of the most difficult for doctors to understand. People who practise the technique do not believe that they are actually doing or applying anything. Indeed, according to them it is not a therapy at all. However, thousands have used the technique and some go as far as to claim that their lives have been transformed by it.

The theory behind it

Adherents of the metamorphic technique (MT) believe that our feet are in some way indicative of the time we spent in the womb, when our characteristics, strengths and weaknesses were first determined. Practitioners claim that by lightly touching areas along an imaginary line (called a 'time line') which runs from the ankle along the arch to the big toe, as well as parts of the hands and head, they can free the person's 'life force', which in turn can alter negative patterns laid down in the past. They feel strongly that they are not the ones doing the healing; they merely act as a catalyst – an agent of change. Touching the feet, hands and head is just 'focusing the consciousness of the body on something to do'; the actual healing is done by the subject himself.

Practitioners use the analogy of a house to describe what they do. In most therapies, the practitioner enters one of the rooms and metaphorically gives it a spring-clean. In MT, all the doors and windows are left open and the fresh air wafting through the house is left to create health and harmony.

What it might be good for

Practitioners do not claim that the technique itself is good for anything – indeed, that is one of the conditions of membership of the
Metamorphic Association* (see below). Only the life force of the
subject can bring about the healing.

People come to practitioners with a variety of conditions,
including cancer and myalgic encephalomyelitis (ME). MT is also
considered to be good for treating addictions because it encourages
a person's 'vital energy' to fight the drugs or alcohol, thus restoring
lost self-esteem. MT seems to be particularly beneficial for people
with long-term physical and mental illnesses.

History

MT was developed in the 1960s by a British naturopath and reflexologist, Robert St John, who worked in an institution for children
with autism and Down's syndrome. He found that his work as a
reflexologist was helpful, but only in the short term. The children
returned to the same old patterns of ill health after treatment. He
formulated the view that the only approach that would work perma-
nently would be the freeing of one's own life force to do the healing.
Gaston Saint-Pierre was taught the technique by St John, and he
went on to establish the Metamorphic Association in 1979.

Treatment

A session usually lasts an hour. The practitioner gently touches the
inside of the foot and hand and the head, in that order, spending
about half an hour on the feet, which are considered more important than the hands or head. He or she will use light stroking
movements, sometimes circular, working perhaps just a few centimetres above the skin.

The practitioner does not ask about your personal life or illnesses, or give advice on diet, lifestyle or anything else. He would
regard that very much as imposing his understanding on you,
which is not part of the MT philosophy. That is why a practitioner
would not even advise you to come again: he would leave it up to
you to make a decision on it. According to practitioners, people

must develop their own authority; if they return for further treatment it will be only because their own 'innate intelligence' directs them to.

Through the metamorphic technique the patient gains inner strength and self-esteem because he or she is the one who is doing the healing and making happen what practitioners call a 'transformation'. This transformation takes place through the life force of the person, either by him changing his approach to how he lives his life, or by seeking what is right for him, such as a change in diet.

After a session with an MT practitioner you should feel very relaxed. A day or so later you may experience a surge of energy or feel a bit confused, which Saint-Pierre says is to be expected, as the mind needs time to adjust to the transformation. Practitioners are very open about the technique, and patients are taught how to use it at home and on their families.

Does it work?

No evidence exists to prove that MT works. Indeed, gathering evidence would be against the whole approach of the technique. Because practitioners believe that people heal themselves, nothing is *done* and therefore nothing can be tested.

Nevertheless, GPs and hospital doctors are showing interest in the technique and a few have practitioners attached to their surgeries and clinics. Some GPs maintain that MT is good for relieving stress and stress-related conditions.

Can it do any harm?

Because the technique is non-invasive, it can do no harm. However, if you have a serious medical condition you should consult your GP first.

How to choose a practitioner

The Metamorphic Association has 150 members. Over 2,000 people have undergone weekend training courses given by Saint-Pierre. The aim of the association is to show people the technique so that they can return home and start using it with family and friends. Through practice they will discover the importance of detachment. As a 'catalyst' the practitioner needs to be completely detached, and that cannot be taught, asserts Saint-Pierre: it has to be experienced. If the practitioner is not detached he will take on the problems of others and become fatigued himself.

Cost

About £25 for an hour, although some practitioners charge less.

NATUROPATHY

AT THE heart of naturopathy is the simple tenet that, given the right set of circumstances, the body, through what naturopaths call its own 'inner vitality', has the power to heal itself. Like many other complementary therapists, naturopaths believe that disease is brought about by an imbalance in the body and that illness affects the whole person – mind, body and spirit – not just an isolated organ.

The theory behind it

The aim of the naturopath is to bring the body back to the point where it can heal itself. This is achieved using various means, including fasting, adjustments to the diet, hydrotherapy and exercise. Practitioners also use osteopathic and chiropractic techniques of manipulation.

Naturopaths are not solely concerned with alleviating symptoms, which in many cases they see as a manifestation of the body's inner vitality fighting off obstructions to its normal functioning. They endeavour to correct the basic causes of disease, starting from the principle that pure water, fresh air, exercise and a balanced diet of fresh foods are the foundations of good health.

Naturopathy has developed in different ways in different parts of the world. European practitioners use more hydrotherapy and herbal medicines, while in the United States naturopaths specialise in herbal and homeopathic treatments and rely on blood and urine tests to form clinical judgements. In the UK practitioners rely on clinical skills, including laboratory tests where necessary, for diagnosis, and treatment is focused on adjustments to the diet, nutritional supplements and herbal medicines.

What it might be good for

The principles of naturopathy can be applied to any disease or condition, though not every patient can be cured. Practitioners claim that chronic conditions such as myalgic encephalomyelitis (ME), constipation, irritable bowel syndrome, eczema, migraine, premenstrual syndrome, allergies, sinusitis, hay fever and asthma respond well to naturopathic treatment.

Many musculo-skeletal ailments can be alleviated by naturopathy as practitioners are skilled in soft-tissue techniques. These techniques include massage and manipulation to ease muscle tension and imbalances. They form part of the naturopath's osteopathic work, which focuses more on gentle stretching than on vigorous mobilising of joints.

History

The roots of naturopathy can be traced back 2,000 years to the Greek physician Hippocrates, who was one of the first to recognise nature's own healing powers - *vis medicatrix naturae*. The ancient Greeks had 'temples of healing', often built near mineral or thermal springs, where patients were put through a regime of bathing, exercise, massage and fasting.

In the eighteenth and nineteenth centuries Europeans began to see the attraction of thermal and spring waters. Coastal towns extolled the virtues of bracing sea walks and sea-bathing, while inland towns boasted of the curative powers of their natural springs. In the UK, for example, Tunbridge Wells had sulphurous water, good for purifying the blood; Bath had hot waters rich in minerals and Epsom was known for its mineral salts. Spas sprang up all over continental Europe – Vichy in France, Baden-Baden in Germany, Marienbad in the Czech Republic. Many of those on the continent are still thriving, but the UK does not have many left.

In the early nineteenth century, Vincent Preissnitz developed a 'water cure' (basically hydrotherapy) in Grafenberg in the mountains of Austrian Silesia, now part of the Czech Republic. He built outdoor baths in the woods where his clients ate a simple diet and drank spring water to cleanse their kidneys and flush out toxins. The treatments they underwent included enemas and plunging alternately into hot and cold baths to stimulate circulation.

This harrowing, yet bracing, regime was enormously popular and soon Preissnitz's 'Water University', as he boldly proclaimed it, was frequented by the upper classes of Europe. In the late 1800s a Bavarian priest, Father Sebastian Kneipp, classified the therapeutic uses of water in *My Water Cure,* still regarded today as a classic text, and throughout Germany there are still centres devoted to *Kneipptherapie.*

In the UK the first residential nature cure resort was set up at Orchard Leigh in 1928 by Stanley Lief. In the early 1930s he moved to larger premises at Champneys, near Tring in Hertfordshire. For many years it was a leading centre of naturopathic healing. Today Tyringham House in Buckinghamshire is the only truly naturopathic clinic in the UK. It offers hydrotherapy, osteopathy, therapeutic fasting, physiotherapy, acupuncture and relaxation techniques – all of which are designed to promote the removal of toxins from the body.

Treatment

An initial consultation with a naturopath will be similar to one with a doctor. Naturopaths undergo training similar to that of doctors and use the same basic diagnostic techniques, although they often place a different interpretation on the results.

The practitioner will take a detailed medical history, feel your pulse, take your blood pressure, listen to your heart and lungs, and look at your posture. But he or she will also question you on your bowel movements, diet, menstrual cycle, work and relationships.

Naturopaths sometimes use the services of a laboratory to analyse body fluids and carry out standard tests, or they will do their own special tests: for instance, to see whether the gut or stomach is working well. If they feel that there is a serious underlying medical problem, you will be referred back to your doctor.

The aim of the naturopath is to evaluate the function of the body. If the patient has good vitality he may respond well to physical measures and diet change. If he is devitalised, more supportive treatment with herbs and nutritional supplements may be needed. Many ailments are the result of poorly functioning organs such as liver, stomach and intestines, often without there being obvious signs of disease in these organs. Some naturopaths use iridology – examination of signs in the eye – as an adjunct to their assessment of the strengths and weaknesses of the different parts of the body.

When the underlying cause of your problem has been diagnosed, the naturopath will draw up a plan for treatment, which will vary according to the condition. The most common proposal is to change the diet: naturopaths claim that most ailments will respond to changes in the diet. All practitioners recommend a diet that is 'biologically aligned', that is, one that includes plenty of fruit, preferably organic, no sugar or refined foods, small amounts of free-range meat and the minimum of alcohol, tea and coffee (and tobacco).

The patient may be asked to keep a diet diary for a few weeks, while the naturopath eliminates certain foods from his diet to see how your body responds. Practitioners say asthma and hay fever seem to respond well to the removal of dairy products from the diet, and that sugar may disturb the biochemistry of the body, thus making it more susceptible to allergic disorders.

Naturopaths sometimes use fasting – controlled abstinence from food – to detoxify the body and treat obesity, allergies, arthritis and rheumatism. The patient could be asked to abstain from food for two or three days and drink nothing but water, or may be allowed fruit or vegetable juices.

Hydrotherapy is central to naturopathy and as part of the treatment the patient may be advised to take hot and cold baths, sometimes filled with epsom salts or seaweed. If the patient has a bronchial condition, he could be advised to apply hot and cold compresses to the chest, throat or abdomen.

The patient may experience what naturopaths call a 'healing crisis' after a few weeks: someone who has chronic bronchitis, for instance, may have a chesty cold and a cough. Or he may experience loose bowels, a rash or a fever. This is regarded as a positive response to treatment and is sometimes enhanced by 'fever' therapy, in which hydrotherapy or herbs are used to raise the body temperature.

Doctors believe illness is caused by germs or viruses from the outside. The naturopathic view is that acute symptoms may sometimes be the expression of the body's efforts to overcome these external agents, and that they should not be suppressed unless they pose a serious threat to the health of people of poor vitality, such as the elderly. Naturopaths would not recommend suppressing an infection associated with a cold with antibiotics, for example, but would encourage the natural resolution of the condition with diet changes, physical therapy and herbs.

Does it work?

One of the main aims of the naturopath is to facilitate the detoxification process. The theory – common to many complementary therapies – is that the body is exposed to a wide variety of potentially harmful compounds present in late twentieth-century society from processed, chemical-laden food, hydrogenated fats, petrol fumes, chemicals sprayed on fruit and vegetables, and hormones in the milk we drink.

People take in so many of these toxins that the liver, which breaks down toxins in the body, is overloaded. Naturopaths believe that a solution is to give the liver and the gastrointestinal tract a rest so that the body will revert to a healthy state and rid itself of disease.

It could be argued that it is no more necessary to rest the liver than to rest the lungs which oxygenate the blood.

Nevertheless, recent research has shown the existence of molecules called free radicals (compounds which invade stable molecules in cell walls, causing damage). They do not have their full complement of electrons and in order to make up this deficiency they try to acquire electrons by reacting with any biological molecule they come across, thereby damaging that molecule and causing damage. Many chronic diseases, including coronary heart disease, are now thought to involve uncontrolled free-radical action.

The job of free radicals is to turn food and oxygen into energy, and in a healthy body they normally disappear within microseconds. But when you have too many of them, through age, illness or external sources such as cigarette smoke or pollution, they can slowly destroy the body.

The latest research shows that a plentiful intake of fresh fruit and vegetables – at least five portions a day – builds up resistance to disease, destroys free radicals and may guard against cancer, coronary heart disease and cataracts.

Several research studies have shown fasting and a vegetarian diet to be effective treatments for patients with rheumatoid arthritis.

Can it do any harm?

The element of naturopathic treatment that causes most concern is fasting. Fasting and special diets need to be professionally supervised. While it might be prudent to eat lightly the day after a heavy business lunch or a celebration dinner, it is not a good idea to cut out food altogether and replace it with a liquid 'diet'.

Fasting does not cleanse the liver. On the contrary, it overworks it by flooding it with toxins caused by not having enough food. Many people who are on 'elimination' diets feel under par and usually have a headache. Most naturopaths say this is a sign that the toxins are being eliminated. However, by fasting you are starving the brain of sugar and your body has to readjust its metabolism and start raiding fat and muscle for sustenance.

How to choose a practitioner

Anyone can call himself a naturopath, set up a naturopathic college or school and establish a register. So make sure that the practitioner who treats you is registered with the General Council and Register of Naturopaths,* which is the only register which requires that its members have completed full-time training.

All of the Register's 220-plus members, identified by the initials MRN (Member of the Register of Naturopaths) after their name, are fully qualified, insured and subject to a strict code of ethics. The majority of registered practitioners are graduates of the four-year full-time course in naturopathy and osteopathy run by the British College of Naturopathy and Osteopathy in London.

Cost

A first consultation will last about an hour and cost £50-£60 in London (£35-£40 outside the capital). Subsequent visits are half as long and cost £25-£30 (less outside London). The number of times you need to see a practitioner depends on the problem – for instance, if you are being treated for a skin problem with herbs and special diets, the naturopath may need to see you every few weeks.

OSTEOPATHY

OSTEOPATHY was the first complementary therapy to be regulated by law; in 1993 the Osteopaths Act was passed, protecting patients from untrained and unauthorised practitioners. Central to the Act is the new General Osteopathic Council (GOsC) which is being established at the time of writing. The Council will replace the existing four voluntary bodies which regulate the activities of osteopaths at present. Once the legislation is fully implemented, in 1999, the GOsC will provide regulation for the whole of the osteopathy profession. In order to be accepted on to its register, all practitioners have to meet a number of requirements. They must hold a recognised qualification such as a degree or diploma in osteopathy; have professional indemnity insurance; and undergo compulsory pre-registration training. Only those practitioners who are registered with the GOsC will be able to call themselves an 'osteopath'.

Since 1993 an increasing number of GPs have been offering osteopathy on the NHS. Their confidence in the therapy has grown as a result of the Osteopaths Act 1993 and the support for osteopathy in the British Medical Association's report *Complementary medicine: new approaches to good practice*, published in 1993. The introduction of fundholding in GP practices has also enabled more doctors to purchase osteopathy for their patients.

Those who use osteopathy seem to be satisfied with the results. An estimated 100,000 people in Britain visit an osteopath every week according to a *Which? Way to Health* survey published in October 1993. In the *Which?* study published in November 1995 (see Appendix), 28 per cent of those respondents who had ever used a complementary therapy had visited an osteopath in the previous 12 months, making it the most widely used therapy among the respondents.

The theory behind it

Osteopaths both diagnose problems and treat the whole person by manipulating the musculo-skeletal system (bones, joints, muscles, ligaments and connective tissues); they believe that when the mechanics of the body are not sound, all sorts of ailments occur. The origin of discomfort or malfunction throughout the body is said to be caused by 'osteopathic lesions' (imbalances in the normal tension of the spine), which affect the nervous system. Osteopaths use a variety of manipulative techniques to correct the underlying cause of pain. These include massage to relax stiff muscles; stretching to help joint mobility; and manipulation and high-velocity thrust techniques, which can restore easy movement to the body. Sometimes osteopaths use 'indirect techniques', particularly on elderly patients and children, which involve light touching and gentle positioning of the joints to reduce tension and restore balance.

The cranial approach is an 'indirect technique' which is based on the idea that there are tiny gaps between the eight sections of the human skull. It is thought that these sections can be pushed out of position (for example, at birth or as a result of a head injury), causing tension, disturbances and tissue immobility not only in the skull but throughout the body. The osteopath will use very gentle manipulation to ease the parts of the skull back into place, thereby correcting the faults.

What it might be good for

Osteopathy is used to treat a variety of musculo-skeletal problems, but 50 per cent of people who visit osteopaths do so to find relief for back pain. Indeed, osteopathy has successfully treated many cases of both chronic and acute back pain where conventional medicine has failed. According to the National Back Pain Association* about 60 per cent of people in Britain will suffer from some form of back pain, brought on by injury, disease, abuse or misuse, at some time in their life. Back problems can be caused by lifting heavy objects in manual occupations, but jobs involving new technology also take their toll; sitting for eight hours with an incorrectly set up work station (i.e. badly adjusted chair, and computer screen placed to the right or left and at the wrong height) can cause back and neck pain.

Osteopathy can be used to ease pain during pregnancy, for asthma, constipation and premenstrual syndrome. It is also used to relieve the symptoms of osteoarthritis. However, it is not appropriate for rheumatoid arthritis, which is an inflammatory disease.

Gentle osteopathy, using the cranial approach, is used for babies with colic, glue ear and sinus problems. Although it is used mainly for children, it can also be used in adults for relieving face, neck and jaw pain, headaches, sinusitis, middle-ear problems and correcting disturbances of the delicate bones and joints of the skull, which might have resulted from injury or trauma.

History

Osteopathy was founded in the 1870s by an American doctor and trained engineer, Andrew Taylor Still. He became convinced that the body could not thrive unless it was structurally sound, and once it was sound, the body's self-healing mechanisms would restore normal function. He coined the term 'osteopathy' from the Greek words *osteo* (meaning 'bone') and *pathos* (meaning 'disease') for his specialised form of treatment. Still set up a school in Kirksville, Missouri, to teach osteopathy. The therapy was then brought over to the UK at the beginning of the twentieth century and the first osteopathy school was set up in London in 1917.

Treatment

On your first visit to an osteopath you will be asked about your medical and life history and any aches and pains. You will then be asked to remove some of your clothing and carry out a series of movements which will enable the practitioner to assess your mobility. Lifestyle factors are also taken into account so that a full diagnosis can be reached – your problems may be the result of a particular sport you do, or bad posture, for example. A suitable treatment plan can then be determined. Subsequent treatment sessions will be taken up with work on the skin, muscles and connective tissue. The osteopath may also use a high-velocity, short and precise 'thrust' technique designed to improve the range of movement of a joint. The sound of this is far worse than the sensation, and you should not feel any pain or discomfort.

Although manipulation forms a major part of osteopathy, osteopaths also advise on remedial exercises to correct postural faults.

Treatment sessions take 30-45 minutes, and osteopaths say that most people get maximum benefit from three to six sessions. They are trained to recognise when a problem is not treatable by osteopathy, for example, if there is evidence of pathology, and will then refer you back to you GP.

Does it work?

Considerable evidence shows that spinal manipulation is of benefit for low back pain. However, in many trials it is not clear which type of practitioner and manipulation was studied. Very few trials exist which explicitly state that osteopathic manipulation was the technique used and no research evidence supports the belief that any one form of manipulation is more effective than any other.

According to *Clinical guidelines for the management of acute low back pain*, published by the Royal College of General Practitioners, manipulative techniques such as osteopathy, chiropractic and manipulative physiotherapy provide short-term improvement in pain, mobility and patient satisfaction within the first six weeks of a back pain episode.

A study published in November 1991 examined the results of 36 randomised clinical trials which compared spinal manipulation with other treatments; it concluded that although the results were promising, the efficacy of manipulation had not been shown convincingly.

A number of scientific studies have looked at whether spinal manipulation is effective in treating low back pain compared with other methods, such as exercises and drug therapy. An American review (1992) of clinical trials of spinal manipulation (on chiropractic and osteopathy) concluded that spinal manipulation was more effective in the treatment of low back pain than other comparable treatments. Researchers considered 58 reports, including results from 25 clinical trials, and came to the conclusion that spinal manipulation was of short-term benefit to some patients, particularly those with uncomplicated, acute low back pain. However, they added that 'data are insufficient concerning the efficacy of spinal manipulation for chronic low back pain'.

Can it do any harm?

If osteopathy is used improperly it can do damage. It is important to give the practitioner a full medical history as there are some conditions which make osteopathy (and its sister therapy, chiropractic) unsuitable:

- recent fractures and whiplash injuries
- osteoporosis (brittle bones)
- pregnancy (during the first three months)
- ankylosing spondylitis (a particular form of inflammation of the joints between the spinal vertebrae)
- cervical or thoracic myelopathy (disease of the spinal cord)
- rheumatoid arthritis.

The most frequent of the reported complications of manipulation of the spine are vascular accidents, which are the crushing or cutting of the veins or arteries, particularly following neck manipulations. However, these are very rare.

Medical papers report 30 deaths from spinal manipulation worldwide since records began, and a number of serious complications have also been reported, including compression of the *cauda equina*, which is a collection of nerve roots at the lower third of the spine. Some people have reported that the pain which they originally went to relieve increased rather than decreased.

However, bearing in mind the number of consultations – in Britain alone it amounts to five million – that are performed each year, the number of recorded complications is extremely low. Since the beginning of the twentieth century, fewer than 200 accidents have been reported while an estimated 6 billion manipulations have been carried out (see Chiropractic for more information).

How to choose a practitioner

Either your GP can refer you to an osteopath under the NHS or you can refer yourself. After 1999 all osteopaths will have to be registered with the GOsC so it will be safe to go to any practitioner on its register. However, until then poorly trained osteopaths are still free to practise under common law. A study carried out in 1992 in England, Scotland and Wales revealed that one in 20 osteopaths, many of whom were trained doctors, physiotherapists or nurses, had no osteopathic qualifications.

Until the GOsC is fully established, check that the practitioner is registered with one of the following: the General Council and Register of Osteopaths (MRO);* the College of Osteopathic Practitioners Association (MCO, FCO);* Natural Therapeutic and Osteopathic Society and Register (MNTOS, FNTOS);* or the Guild of Osteopaths (MGO, FGO).* Membership of one of these organisations means that the practitioner is insured, works to a code of ethics and is bound by a disciplinary procedure. The initials in brackets appear after the practitioners' name if they are members. Also check that the practitioner has trained at an approved college (the British School of Osteopathy, the British College of Naturopathy and Osteopathy, or the European School of Osteopathy). The London College of Osteopathic Medicine runs a 13-month full-time post-graduate course for doctors; it awards an MLCOM (membership qualification) or a FLCOM (fellowship). All qualified osteopaths have either DO or BSc (Ost) after their name, indicating a diploma or degree in osteopathy.

Contact the Osteopathic Information Service* for a list of members of these organisations in your area.

Cost

The first consultation will cost anything from £25 (outside London) up to £60 (in London). Subsequent sessions will cost anything from £18 to £30 (or possibly more in London). Some private health insurance companies will pay for osteopathic treatment, so check whether your policy covers it. You can have osteopathic treatment under the NHS if your doctor is willing to refer you.

Radiesthesia and Radionics

MANY people find it difficult to take radiesthesia and radionics seriously. These therapies involve pendulums, hazel twigs, strange, quasi-scientific, electric instruments – some not even plugged in – and healing energy waves emitted from some distant clinic. It is not necessary to meet your practitioner face to face; instead you send him or her a body sample – usually hair or a drop of blood – with the help of which a diagnosis will then be made.

The theory behind them

According to advocates of radiesthesia and radionics, all matter emits radiation, which can be studied, measured and interpreted in order to make a medical diagnosis.

Practitioners of radiesthesia apply techniques similar to those used in dowsing or water-divining. Dowsers walk over a piece of ground carrying two metal rods or a forked, hazel twig. When they cross a buried well or stream, the twig dips, indicating the spot.

A medical dowser or radiesthetist (from the French *radiesthésie*, meaning 'dowsing') uses a pendulum instead of a dowser's twig. He or she works from a sample or 'witness' of the patient, usually a strand of hair, nail clipping or spot of blood on a filter paper, hangs a pendulum over it and observes whether it swings clockwise or anti-clockwise or to and fro.

The practitioner may then hold the witness in one hand and with the other hand dangle the pendulum over a range of medications, probably herbal and homeopathic. The pendulum will indicate which one is the correct choice for that specific ailment.

What they might be good for

Practitioners claim that radiesthesia and radionics can help stress, asthma, hay fever and other allergies, musculo-skeletal problems and digestive ailments. Generally, they improve energy, they assert, by removing 'blockages'. Animals, which are treated in the same way as humans, are supposed to respond well, as are crops. Indeed, some practitioners specialise in the treatment of soil and crops and maintain that these therapies are natural methods of weed and pest control.

History

Medical dowsing became popular at the turn of the century. Two French priests, the Abbés Bouley and Mermet, developed considerable expertise in using a pendulum for dowsing and Abbé Mermet wrote *Principles and Practice of Radiesthesia* (1959), which contained records of his results over a 40-year period.

The Medical Society for the Study of Radiesthesia was founded in Britain in 1939. One of its members, a surgeon called George Laurence, postulated a link between radiesthetic diagnoses and homeopathic remedies.

Radionics is basically radiesthesia with machines. The principles of radionics were described early this century by an American neurologist, Albert Abrams. He argued that radiation is a universal property of matter (a novel idea at the time) and that the basis of disease, being electronic rather than cellular, could be reflected in its radiations. The word 'radionics' is an amalgam of 'radiation' and 'electronics'.

Abrams discovered that the sound made by tapping (percussing) a patient's body varies according to the area percussed and the nature of the disease. He later found that he could obtain the same note when a healthy person held diseased tissue in his or her hand.

He invented a 'black box' – the clinical equivalent of a radio receiving set – to pick up radiations from diseased tissue which could then be diagnosed and treated via the same piece of machinery. The patient, or even a spot of blood, could be linked via an electrode to the box. He leased the box out to anybody who would pay the tuition fees and a $300 charge.

After Abrams's death in 1924 an American chiropractor, Dr Ruth Drown, developed his work and designed a new instrument. In 1950 the American Medical Association's learned journal reported on an investigation carried out on her instrument at the University of Chicago. She was given ten blood specimens to analyse, but her diagnoses of the first three were so inaccurate that she did not proceed with the tests. She was later convicted of quackery and fraud by the US Food and Drug Administration.

In Britain, the engineer George de la Warr took up radionics in the 1950s. In 1960 he established the Radionic Association* as a limited company. He invented his own instruments, including a 'camera' that took a 'photograph' of a person's internal organs when a spot of his or her blood was inserted into the device.

None of these instruments connected up to anything or was plugged in, apart from to the patient or the blood spot. When a dissatisfied operator who had bought one of de la Warr's instruments sued him, in 1960, the judge was sceptical about the instrument, but was satisfied that de la Warr honestly believed it to work and therefore did not consider him to be doing anything fraudulent.

Treatment

Radionics can be used to diagnose people, animals and plants. You may not see the practitioner, but will be sent a detailed case-history form to fill in. Most practitioners will ask for a small snippet of your hair or a drop of blood on a piece of blotting paper. They do not analyse this 'witness', but use it as a 'connecting' link between the patient, instrument and practitioner.

The practitioner will then 'tune in' to the patient via the witness and make an analysis of his health, assessing the physical, emotional, spiritual and mental states, balance of energy and predisposition to major diseases. He or she will establish what treatment is necessary.

This is normally done by directing 'corrective' energy to the patient via the hair or blood spot. Instruments are used to establish the energy strength and wavelength. Sometimes the practitioner uses other complementary techniques, such as acupuncture, homeopathy or herbal medicine, in addition.

Some practitioners now link patients to a computer which will automatically produce a diagnosis and suggest treatment.

Do they work?

Most doctors are highly sceptical about radiesthesia and radionics, for which no scientific evidence exists to back up practitioners' claims.

In 1936 the University of Hanover invited practitioners of radiesthesia to diagnose 19 animals. After comparing diagnoses made conventionally and by radiesthesia, scientists found the latter were both wrong and inconsistent. Moreover, healthy animals were diagnosed as being ill. In 1992, another German study showed that there was no scientific proof of the validity of the technique.

Can they do any harm?

On the face of it, radionics and radiesthesia cannot cause harm, but some practitioners believe that they can be used for 'evil' as well as good purposes. Some of the techniques of radionics resemble those of witch-doctors and magicians, particularly in its use of hair and blood spots. Some practitioners believe that the therapies can be used to manipulate the mind without the knowledge of its owner.

But how hair strands, which we all shed indiscriminately every day, can be used for evil purposes, or a mind controlled from possibly several hundred miles away, is beyond scientists – and, indeed, most rational minds.

How to choose a practitioner

The Radionic Association is the main organisation in the field, with its own School of Radionics. It takes about 18 months of part-time study to qualify as a licentiate of the Association and a further 18 months to qualify as a full member. Pupils who qualify are entitled to put MRadA (Member of the Radionic Association) after their name. A list of qualified members is available from the Association for a small fee.

Cost

About £25 for the analysis, plus £25 for subsequent monthly treatments.

REFLEXOLOGY

REGARDLESS of whether a reflexologist balances energy levels or stimulates various organs, the very act of having your feet massaged is calming. Practitioners claim that it is beneficial to health too, and with an increasing number of reflexologists being employed in hospitals, orthodox medicine seems to be starting to take this therapy seriously.

The theory behind it

Reflexology, or reflex zone therapy as it is sometimes called, is a treatment in which the practitioner applies pressure to the feet or (less commonly) the hands in order to assess the health of the patient and promote well-being. Zone therapy divides the body into ten vertical zones which run from the feet up the body to the head and down to the hands, and through which flows energy.

Practitioners believe that all the body's organs, systems and parts are reflected in the feet. By massaging the reflexes, the therapist stimulates the corresponding organs in the body, releasing natural healing powers and restoring a state of health. For instance, the sinuses are 'located' at the top of the toes, so working in this area should ease a stuffy nose. Experienced reflexologists claim they can detect and even relieve a bladder problem, say, by putting pressure on the corresponding part of the foot.

Some reflexologists believe that crystalline deposits of calcium and uric acid build up at the nerve endings and feel 'crunchy' under the skin. They claim that if they feel a slight swelling, lump or 'squidginess', this could indicate a weakness in a specific area of the body. Gentle pressure on these deposits is thought to break them down and begin the healing process.

This healing takes place via 'energy pathways', which according to reflexologists can become blocked and prevent the body from working effectively. Reflexology can be used to clear these pathways and maintain the energy balance. Some practitioners believe that these pressure points are the same as acupuncture points and that the energy pathways are meridians (see Acupuncture).

What it might be good for

Practitioners claim that reflexology can bring about a general improvement in energy levels and emotional well-being. Unlike acupuncture or homeopathy, the code of ethics of the Association of Reflexologists* (one of the major organisations in the field; see below) states that members should not diagnose medical conditions, prescribe treatment, or claim they can cure any specific ailment.

Reflexology has been used to alleviate migraine, headaches, back problems and stress-related conditions. Practitioners believe that it can also help asthma, skin disorders such as eczema and psoriasis, high blood pressure, poor circulation, constipation and irritable bowel syndrome.

Even if there is no immediate improvement in the condition for which treatment is sought, therapists maintain that people benefit from fully relaxing, talking or being silent in the presence of someone whose full attention is on them. This could be said about many complementary therapies. Just lying down for an hour, being touched and letting someone else take control is deeply soothing. As such, it can hardly not ease tension and tension-related conditions.

History

Evidence has shown that hand and foot massage was used in India and China over 5,000 years ago, but in 1913 Dr William Fitzgerald, an American surgeon, found that pressure on particular parts of the hand and foot could cause partial anaesthesia to areas of the ear, nose and throat. By using these pressure points, Dr Fitzgerald

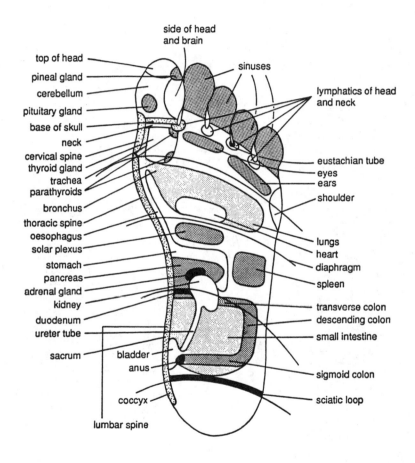

Figure 4 The reflexes on the left foot as seen from underneath

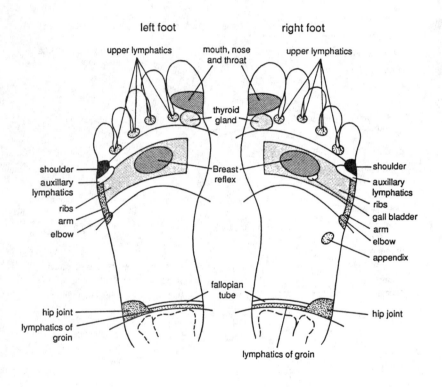

Figure 5 The reflexes on top of the feet

claimed he could perform minor surgery without conventional anaesthetics. He put forward the idea that the body is divided into ten equal vertical zones, and that pressure on one part of a zone could affect every other part of that zone.

The idea was popularised in the 1930s by the American physiotherapist Eunice Ingham, who devised her own method of foot massage. Doreen Bayley, a student of Ingham, introduced reflexology to the UK, and in 1968 set up the Bayley School of Reflexology.

Treatment

Each session lasts about an hour. The reflexologist will want to know about your medical history and lifestyle, whether you are taking any medication and whether you have come for treatment of any particular condition. You will be invited to lie down on a couch or reclining chair with your bare feet raised. Do not worry if your feet are hot and sweaty, as the practitioner will wipe them before starting.

The practitioner works over all areas of the feet, either moving from one foot to the other or working on each foot separately. Initially, gentle massage is used, followed by deep thumb and finger pressure. If the practitioner feels that an imbalance or blockage is present, the part of the foot which corresponds to the affected body part may feel tender. Gentle pressure is used to remove the blockage. It can be sensitive, though not unbearably so, and a first-time client will usually be treated gently.

Most people feel relaxed after treatment, but some may feel sleepy or light-headed. Some have reported 'flu-like symptoms, feeling cold for three to four days afterwards or wanting to go to the lavatory more frequently.

Does it work?

A good deal of anecdotal evidence suggests that reflexology does work, and there is no doubt that it can relieve stress. But, as with many therapies, few scientific data have been produced to back up the experiences of reflexology's devotees, or to confirm the existence of zones, energy lines or crystalline deposits.

Nevertheless, doctors are aware that internal organs are represented on the surface of the area of skin that is served by the same nerves as the organs. In addition, pain sensations which may arise in one part of the body may be relieved by stimulating the foot, simply because the nerves both from the foot and from the affected body part converge on the same cells in the spinal cord. Reflexology may close the 'sensory gate', thus preventing pain signals from reaching the brain.

Many small research studies attest to its benefits. In 1993, an American reflexologist, Bill Flocco, carried out a six-month trial on 35 women suffering from premenstrual syndrome. Fifty per cent were given reflexology, and 50 per cent had what they thought was reflexology but was in fact just foot massage.

The women recorded how they felt with respect to 39 different physical and psychological symptoms every day for six menstrual cycles and rated them on a four-point scale: none, mild, moderate and strong. The results showed that of those having reflexology, 39 per cent experienced an improvement, whereas of those who thought they were having reflexology but were not, only 13.8 per cent felt that their condition had improved.

Reflexology seems to be particularly beneficial for people suffering from cancer and undergoing radiotherapy and chemotherapy; studies are under way in the cancer units at Charing Cross and Hammersmith Hospitals, London, and the Queen Elizabeth Hospital, Birmingham, to see how cancer patients respond to reflexology. Each patient is offered four sessions during the course of chemotherapy.

The therapy is not used to *cure* cancer, but to help patients relax, improve their quality of life and help them cope with the anxiety created by their illness and the side-effects of their treatment – insomnia, constipation, nausea, needle phobia and pain.

The projects at the hospitals have the support of all medical staff. The reflexologists working there report that according to the patients the only time they do not think about their disease is when they are having reflexology. The therapy helps relieve tension and therefore pain; having their feet massaged is by far the most pleasant experience the patients have in hospital.

Can it do any harm?

Although reflexology is in no way harmful, nurses are taught that it should be used with care when dealing with people who have epilepsy, or who are depressed. Some reflexologists are reluctant to treat people with diabetes or thyroid problems, or pregnant women, but there are no data to show that reflexology is harmful in these or any other cases.

If a reflexologist suspects from an assessment of the feet that there may be a serious underlying condition, he or she should advise you to go to your GP, in accordance with the professional code of ethics and practice.

How to choose a practitioner

In 1989 the Association of Reflexologists, in collaboration with a number of schools, formed a working party to set standards for the training of professional reflexologists. The Association has now accredited nearly 70 courses in the UK which meet its standards. The British Reflexology Association,* founded in 1985, is the professional organisation associated with the Bayley School. Qualified reflexologists can be identified by the initials MAR (Member of the Association of Reflexologists) or MBRA (Member of the British Reflexology Association).

Both organisations have codes of practice and ethics, and therapists must have insurance. A list of local accredited therapists is available from either organisation.

Cost

About £20-£30, depending on where the practitioner is based.

ROLFING

ROLFING, named after its inventor Dr Ida Rolf, an American biochemist, is also known as 'structural integration'. It is a system of physical manipulation and postural release which aims to loosen up the body and realign it.

The theory behind it

Rolfers believe that our bodies are in constant battle with the pull of gravity, a condition which is exasperated by the strains and stresses of life. Poor posture affects our emotional and physical well-being. A 'disorganised' body expends more energy in remaining upright and becomes tired sooner because it uses energy less efficiently than a body with good posture.

During periods of stress our breathing becomes shallow, the muscles of the abdomen contract and we may tighten the muscles of the shoulders, neck and jaw. Eventually they begin to ache, a sign that there is not enough blood in the muscles. Chronic, long-term tension eventually causes the network of fibrous connective tissue (fascia) covering and linking the muscles to shorten.

Rolfing is designed to lengthen and release the fascia, which in turn is said to improve blood flow and eliminate energy loss caused by muscle strain. Once you have been 'rolfed' it might look as though you are just standing a bit straighter, but rolfers say their technique does not just improve posture. The lengthening of the fascia allows the body to re-align itself with gravity, helping the individual to function better. Once this has been achieved, our natural powers of healing can work unimpeded. A 'rolfed' body is at ease, supported by gravity rather than 'at war' with it.

What it might be good for

Rolfing does not claim to cure disease, but practitioners say it can alleviate musculo-skeletal problems, such as bad backs, constipation, period pains, anxiety and stress. Many people say they feel more supple after a rolfing session.

History

In the 1930s, as result of family illness, Dr Ida Rolf began to investigate the causes of poor posture. After spending over 50 years studying bodily structure in thousands of people, she came to the conclusion that chronic poor posture was caused by shortened connective tissue around the muscles and that physical efficiency was at its peak when the major segments of the body – head, shoulders, abdomen, pelvis and legs – were aligned and balanced in a specific way. According to Dr Rolf, the angle of the pelvis is the keystone to integrating the body's weight, and the 'standing pelvic tilt' can be measured by looking at the distances between the tip of the tailbone (coccyx), the front of the pubic bone and the upper part of the pelvis. She discovered that skilful manipulation could lengthen shortened tissue.

Her system eventually became known as the Rolf Method of Structural Integration. In the early 1960s, in response to demand, she began to teach her technique. She visited Britain regularly, teaching her techniques to osteopaths. Today, about 700 practitioners carry on her work throughout the world.

Treatment

Treatment usually consists of ten weekly one-hour sessions. The practitioner will take a case history at the first session, and may take a photograph or video of you from the front, back and sides for analysis later. You may be asked to stand in front of a mirror and try to look at your body through the eyes of the rolfer. As with osteopathy and chiropractic, you will be asked to undress down to your underwear. Then, while you lie on a massage couch, the practitioner will apply pressure with his or her fingers, hands, knuckles or elbows to smooth out the muscles' connective tissues.

Each session will focus on a different part of the body. In the first session, for instance, the practitioner might concentrate on the shoulders, chest, lower back and pelvis; in the second he or she might focus on the area from the knees to the feet, and so on. This is not a particularly relaxing experience – it is sometimes uncomfortable, even painful. After a session you will feel lighter and walk taller as the head and chest lift up and the trunk lengthens. You may actually get taller (about 1 cm), simply because you are holding yourself correctly. But you may feel a bit sore for a few days. Some people experience renewed vigour; others have reported that they sensed an emotional release, feeling the treatment break down long-term stress and tension.

Rolfing has a reputation for being painful, though rolfers say it is no more painful than a deep massage. They say there may be pain as the fascia is released, but this should last only a few seconds and will stop when the rolfing stops.

Does it work?

In 1988 researchers carried out a study on the effects of the soft tissue manipulation used in rolfing on 32 men, each of whom had a slightly forward-tilting pelvis. The group was divided at random and 16 men underwent a 45-minute rolfing session, while the control group received no manipulation.

When the two groups were compared 24 hours later, the men who had undergone rolfing showed a decrease or significant improvement in the angle of tilt of their pelvis and an increase in the activity of the parasympathetic nervous system. The researchers concluded that in this small study the reduction in the pelvic tilt supports the use of rolfing for treatment for certain types of lower back disorders and the increase in activity of the parasympathetic nervous system supports its use in musculo-skeletal dysfunctions associated with reduced parasympathetic nervous activity.

Much of the above could probably be achieved by undergoing Alexander technique or osteopathy.

Can it do any harm?

Rolfing is painful but the rolfer should take care to work within the client's limits. People who have experienced severe emotional trauma should approach rolfing with caution. It is not appropriate for people who bruise very easily or people who are obese.

How to choose a practitioner

Unlike other complementary therapies which have been imported from the United States, rolfing has not established a firm foothold in the UK. There are only nine certified rolfers in the UK at the time of writing.

Cost

About £50 for a 1½-hour session (ten sessions are usually needed).

SHIATSU

SHIATSU, a Japanese word meaning 'finger massage', is a therapy which has its roots in traditional Chinese medicine. Like acupuncture, shiatsu works by stimulating the body's vital energy, *qi* (pronounced 'chee'), which circulates around the body via the meridians, or energy lines (see Acupuncture). The therapy was almost unheard of in the UK until the 1970s, but now about 100 teachers, 81 of whom belong to the Shiatsu Society,* offer treatment.

The theory behind it

Shiatsu works on the principle that disease is caused by a disturbance in the flow of energy through the body: it is depleted (*kyo*), or blocked or over-active (*jitsu*). However deep the problem, it manifests itself on the surface of the body, at points called *tsubos*, via tributaries from the main channel of each meridian. A shiatsu specialist can access the meridian by applying pressure at these points (the same points as are used in acupuncture) using thumbs, fingers, elbows and even knees or feet. He or she may also move and position the body in a way that stretches the meridians.

A do-it-yourself variety of shiatsu called *do-in*, which means 'self-stimulation', is also taught.

What it might be good for

Practitioners claim that shiatsu is good for musculo-skeletal problems, particularly lower back and neck problems. Because it eases muscular tension and stiffness, it is also said to relieve stress. It can be performed on wheelchair-users and can therefore be used for the relief of cerebral palsy and other physical disabilities. Some practitioners work in the NHS on cancer wards and in alcohol and drug rehabilitation centres, while others offer their services to people with HIV and AIDS.

History

Shiatsu developed at the turn of the twentieth century from *anma*, a part of traditional Japanese medicine that has existed for about 2,000 years. Originally used to treat specific conditions, it gradually developed into a form of relaxation. The Japanese government recognises shiatsu as an effective therapy. It is enormously popular in Japan and is becoming more so in Europe and the United States. It was introduced to the UK in the late 1970s, and the Shiatsu Society was formed in 1981.

Treatment

Shiatsu practitioners work on the floor and through clothes, so if you attend a session it is advisable to wear baggy garments, such as a tracksuit. You will probably be told to have only a light meal and to avoid alcohol before the treatment.

The first session will last about 1½ hours. The therapist will begin by taking a case history. As with all types of Oriental medicine (see Acupuncture for details), for the diagnosis the practitioner will ask you about your lifestyle, medical history and symptoms. He will observe your posture, the sparkle in your eyes and the sheen in your hair, and listen to your voice. He may also take your pulse in the traditional Chinese way. Then you will probably be asked remove your shoes and lie down (on a thick mat or futon) for the final stage of diagnosis, which is the *hara*: the practitioner will gently palpate the abdomen to assess the energy flow in the meridians and internal organs.

The treatment itself usually begins with the practitioner stretching, squeezing and turning parts of your body to correct any structural imbalance and release energy blockages. Pressure will then be applied to the *tsubos* using the thumbs or other fingers, or more unusually elbows, knees or feet. This may be slightly painful, but shiatsu will leave you feeling refreshed.

While you will usually experience a feeling of well-being, practitioners say there may be 'healing' reactions. These could take the form of a headache or 'flu-like symptoms for 24 hours. You may experience side-effects such as aches and pains for a day or two.

You will usually be given advice on diet and lifestyle. Therapists say that rather than curing illness, they encourage patients to take charge of and improve their health through a regime of exercises and dietary changes. For help with a specific health or emotional problem, weekly sessions over a period of four to six weeks or longer are recommended. Otherwise, one session a month is enough.

Does it work?

While shiatsu can bring relief to certain groups of people, it has not been the subject of any scientific study. The Shiatsu Society conducted a survey among shiatsu clients, who were asked whether they found the treatment 'very effective', 'effective', 'neutral', 'ineffective' or 'very ineffective'. Of the respondents, 54 per cent found it to be 'very effective' and a further 38 per cent said it was 'effective'. Most used shiatsu for stress and musculo-skeletal disorders, such as back and neck pain.

A study conducted by the Society in 1992 used shiatsu on people with thalamic pain, a rare chronic syndrome caused by damage to the thalamus, the part of the brain that deals with sensations. The pain arising from this disorder, usually caused by a stroke or brain tumour, is often intense and difficult to relieve by orthodox means.

This small study was set up by a teacher of dance who had suffered from thalamic pain for ten years. In 1990 the only drug that gave her relief was withdrawn from the market. This, together with the unpleasant side-effects she experienced from another drug, drove her to try shiatsu to ease the pain. She experienced a dramatic improvement in her condition, which she has maintained.

Seven people with thalamic pain, aged between 50 and 85, took part in the study. They all found painkillers ineffective, but five of them tried shiatsu and three continued to use it after three months. They said that it helped them relax and manage their pain better.

Can it do any harm?

The technique itself is very safe, and the Shiatsu Society says that it has never received a complaint about the treatment. Older people may find it a problem to lie down on the floor, but the technique is adaptable and can be used on someone in a chair or wheelchair. Shiatsu is not used on those with osteoporosis (brittle bones) or on women in the first three months of pregnancy.

How to choose a practitioner

Check that the therapist is a Member of the Register of the Shiatsu Society (MRSS) and conforms to its code of practice and ethics. If he or she is not, there are no means of legal redress in the event of inappropriate behaviour.

Cost

About £20-£30 per session.

T'AI CHI

WESTERNERS visiting China in the early 1970s (the first time in decades they could travel freely there) were entranced to see parks full of people at the crack of dawn exercising as if in a slow-motion film, making gentle, careful movements. Now nearly every adult education institute in the UK has a t'ai chi class, and the practice has thousands of adherents in the West. It is easy to see its attraction; with its beautiful, dance-like movements, t'ai chi is the antithesis of our modern, hurried world.

The theory behind it

T'ai chi, or *t'ai chi chuan* (*t'ai chi* means 'the supreme unity' and *chuan* the 'fist' or 'container'), to give it its full name, comprises a series of postures linked by gentle, graceful movements into forms, which are designed to bring health and well-being by restoring the natural flow of energy within the body.

T'ai chi is influenced by Taoist, Confucian and Buddhist philosophies, which teach that the world is an interplay of two opposing forces, *yin* and *yang*. The movements are a way of stabilising these fluctuating energies and are seen as reflecting the ebb and flow of life. To maintain a state of flow, therapeutic exercises were developed, inspired by the natural movements of nature – the wind, birds in flight, the sea. Kung-fu is the most vigorous of these exercises and is now regarded as a martial art. T'ai chi is a form of kung-fu. It is a martial art, but has been called a 'non-violent martial art', as it has no competitive edge and is usually practised alone.

Qi gong, another exercise, encompasses posture, breathing and focusing the mind. It aims to strengthen the internal energy, or *qi*.

What it might be good for

The concentration and discipline needed to remember the forms still the mind, and the steady breathing calms, de-stresses and focuses each individual. It therefore helps to make one more alert.

This gentle form of exercise is suitable for people with disabilities such as multiple sclerosis and polio, and for those recovering from illness or injuries. Although it is usually performed standing, it can be adapted for wheelchair-users, who gain much benefit from it.

History

Exercising for health has always been a traditional part of Chinese culture, in which an active, but peaceful, mind is assumed to be as necessary to health as a fit, well-toned body. Long before this was widely acknowledged in the West, the Chinese knew that mind and body are inextricably linked, and that tension, anxiety, irritation and fear can interfere with the efficient working of the body.

T'ai chi was developed in the twelfth century, out of kung-fu, by Chang San-feng, a soldier and mystic who was concerned about the hard and aggressive nature of the army's martial training. Having deserted, he spent several years working out the new movements as a long form of kung-fu for fuller spiritual development.

Five main styles of t'ai chi are practised: *yang*, *wu*, *chen*, *woo* and *sun*. Each differs in the kinds of postures and rhythms. The *yang* style, for example, uses large, open gestures, while the *chen* style uses rapid, coiling movements, interspersed with slower ones.

T'ai chi is now practised by millions in China and is increasingly popular in the West. It was introduced into the UK in the 1970s.

Practice

It is best to learn t'ai chi in a class, for two reasons. First, you need someone to demonstrate the movements, and second, it will take you some time to learn them (between six months and three years to gain any proficiency and very much longer to master the movements completely). However, with a good teacher subtle benefits can be experienced after a few lessons.

The 'short form' of t'ai chi consists of movements that can be performed in about ten minutes; the 'long form' takes 20–40 minutes. The movements are slow, pleasurable and linked, so that one flows into another. Although not all t'ai chi practitioners talk in terms of the number of movements, there are over 100 to be learnt. T'ai chi is harder to master than yoga, because you have to remember the movements, but if you have a tendency to forget, or if someone else in the class is 'better' at it than you are, do not get ruffled: you are not in competition with anyone.

Does it work?

Some doctors recommend t'ai chi to patients who have heart problems and high blood pressure. Most people enjoy it and say it makes them feel peaceful and relaxed. As in yoga, many of the movements are aimed at making one more aware of one's own body and its energy, and this in itself gives many people an inner confidence.

Studies have shown that t'ai chi appears to be of benefit in improving balance and cardiovascular function in older people.

Can it do any harm?

T'ai chi is a very gentle form of exercise with no harmful side-effects and many benefits.

How to choose a practitioner

Many local authorities, local adult evening classes and health clubs offer t'ai chi lessons.

Cost

About £5 a class. Some t'ai chi schools run drop-in classes, but you need to have a course of at least ten sessions to get any benefit.

YOGA

ANYONE who has practised yoga (from the Sanskrit word for 'union') knows how relaxing it can be. You might feel tired when you go to a class but, despite putting yourself into physically demanding positions, it is likely that you will feel refreshed and energised after a session. Many people find that after they have been practising regularly for some time, they achieve a mental and emotional calm which spills into their daily lives.

The theory behind it

Yoga postures tone the body, develop the respiratory system, oxygenate the blood and keep the spine strong. Most people in the UK who practise yoga use it to maintain suppleness and to build stamina, without thinking about the philosophy behind it, but it does not have to be just a series of exercises. It can also be a spiritual and mental discipline which combines posture exercises with breath control and meditation to help students achieve mental clarity, spiritual awareness and inner peace. Many varieties of this ancient discipline have been developed over the years. *Hatha* yoga, in which mental and spiritual health is achieved through mastery of the body, is the best-known in the West. Iyengar yoga, a form of *hatha* yoga developed by B.K.S. Iyengar, is the most commonly practised form in the UK.

What it might be good for

Yoga is good for keeping fit and supple and is beneficial for a wide range of ailments. It is particularly good for back pain, and many yoga exercises have been incorporated into general exercise classes. Back rolls, for example, stretch the lower back and massage the spine.

Both postures and breathing exercises can help respiratory disorders such as asthma, hay fever, bronchitis, sinusitis, colds and coughs. Asthma sufferers tend to have shallow breathing, and yoga deepens the breath and induces relaxation, which dissipates any tension which might lead to an attack. Relaxation, deep breathing and postures that massage the inner organs can aid digestion and alleviate digestive disorders such as ulcers and irritable bowel syndrome.

Yoga is also beneficial for people with disabilities. Disability is often exacerbated by lack of exercise and muscles become weak if they are not used, which can lead to further disability and weakening of the joints. There is growing recognition in the West that yoga and t'ai chi provide many of the important elements of exercise for disabled people. They also allow people to become more aware of their bodies and how they move. Mobility is improved not only by greater strength but by greater efficiency and awareness of the body. Much of the work of the Yoga for Health Foundation* is focused on the way in which yoga can help people with multiple sclerosis and other neuro-muscular diseases.

History

Yoga probably existed in some form in India over 5,000 years ago. It was introduced to England in the Victorian era, but became really popular only in the 1960s.

Practice

Yoga is suitable for anyone of any age: you do not have to be a lithe-limbed 20-year-old to benefit. It is best to join a class to learn the postures, then, if you like, you can practise at home. Classes range from slow, meditative sessions through to dynamic and physically taxing forms of yoga. It is unwise to try to learn from a video alone.

The yoga *asanas* (postures), along with the *pranayama* (breathing exercises), are designed to calm the mind and improve the flow of *prana*, or vital energy. The concept of *prana* is very much like the Chinese idea of *qi* (see Acupuncture). *Prana* flows along invisible channels called *nadis*, and poor health is supposedly caused by blockages in these channels. According to yogic tradition, the body has seven major *chakras* (points of focused energy) which are invigorated through yoga. These are found at the crown of the head, the throat, the solar plexus, the spine, the centre of the forehead (the third eye, or brow *chakra*), the heart and the navel. Each *chakra* has certain positive and negative qualities. For instance, the brow *chakra* vitalises the lower brain and central nervous system and is connected with the functioning of the pituitary gland, left eye, nose and ears. Its positive qualities are intuition, concentration, wisdom and peace of mind. Its negative qualities are fear, tension, nightmares and headaches. Meditation, sometimes known as *samayama*, is also a central part of yoga.

A yoga class lasts a minimum of an hour; usually they are 1½-2 hours long. Wear loose-fitting clothing, and remember to take a jumper or sweatshirt; when you are relaxing and meditating at the end of the session, you may feel chilly.

Yoga postures

There are about 80 major postures, but most people practise only about 20. They are performed standing, kneeling, sitting or lying on the front or back. For each *asana* there is a 'counter' *asana* which works in the opposite direction in a less vigorous way. This helps to maintain physiological and mental balance. Many *asanas* work on the spine to keep it strong and supple, while others are said to massage internal organs or act on trigger points in much the same way as acupuncture. The exercises are very precise and, to get the full benefit, instructions must be followed carefully.

Classes usually start with stretching exercises, and *asanas* are interspersed with deep relaxation and breathing exercises. Nearly all classes end with the most famous relaxation posture, *savasna* (the corpse pose), one of yoga's most powerful weapons against stress. When practising yoga, do not force yourself into a position if it feels uncomfortable and do not hold it for too long. Never hurry yoga positions or strain to achieve them.

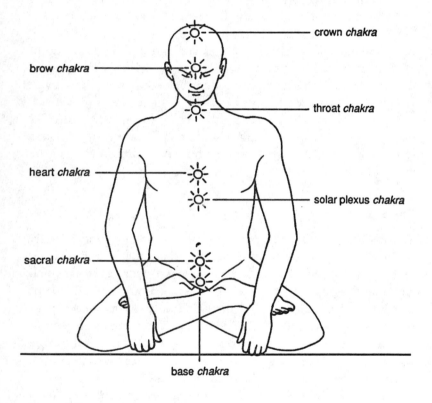

Figure 6 The major *chakras*

Does it work?

There is no doubt that yoga is beneficial for certain conditions. It seems that regular yoga reduces stress, and studies have shown that it can play a part in the management of high blood pressure, heart conditions, asthma and mild forms of diabetes.

In 1983, the Yoga Biomedical Trust* investigated the reactions of 3,000 people who practised yoga and were suffering from one or more of 19 ailments. Of a total of 1,142 suffering from back pain, 98 per cent said their condition had been alleviated by yoga; and of 834 people suffering from symptoms of anxiety, 94 per cent said their symptoms had eased.

In a study in India, 53 people with asthma were taught yoga postures and breathing exercises over a fortnight and were told to practise these exercises every day for 65 minutes. They were compared with a control group which continued to take its usual medication. The results showed that a significantly greater improvement occurred in the symptoms among the group which practised yoga than in the group which stuck to its medication. This is borne out by anecdotal reports at the Yoga Biomedical Trust. The trust trains yoga teachers to work with people who have asthma, chronic fatigue syndrome, diabetes, backache and those who are terminally ill. It claims that yoga can bring relief to people with asthma within three weeks.

It is also possible that yoga is beneficial for non-insulin-dependent diabetics. In another recent study, 21 patients with non-insulin-dependent diabetes mellitus were divided into two groups. All patients continued their medication and special diet, but ten were offered yoga classes, comprising a mixture of postural, breathing and relaxation exercises. Most group members attended twice a week and practised at least once a week at home. After three months the yoga group found that they were able to reduce their drugs and reported feeling better, less anxious and more in control of themselves.

Can it do any harm?

Yoga is not an easy option. Some forms of yoga, such as *ashtanga*, are for the young and healthy, and it would be extremely unwise to attempt a session if you have not exercised regularly for some time.

Forcing your body into a posture or holding it longer than is bearable is inadvisable.

How to choose a teacher

If you have an ailment such as severe backache or diabetes, you can be treated by a yoga therapist on a one-to-one basis. There are about 30 such therapists in the UK, most of them based in London and all are members of the Yoga Biomedical Trust. They run classes for small groups of people, or individuals.

Most people who practise yoga join a local class, run at lunchtime or in the evening in local community premises such as church halls. Make sure the teacher is a member of the British Wheel of Yoga★ or the Iyengar Yoga Institute.★ Some companies now offer lunchtime yoga classes to help employees who suffer from stress, or back and neck pain.

Cost

You can be referred under the NHS by your GP for yoga therapy, but more usually you will have to attend privately, which costs £30 an hour for individual treatment, and between £6 and £12 for a class lasting 90 minutes. For general classes run by a local authority expect to pay between £3 and £5 per class.

ALTERNATIVE MEDICINE SURVEY RESULTS

Consumers' Association conducted a survey of its members (i.e. subscribers to its magazines) in August 1995 to look at various aspects of the usage of complementary (referred to as 'alternative') medicine. The research, the results of which were published in the November 1995 issue of *Which?*, sought information on members' experiences of using practitioners of alternative medicines and their levels of satisfaction with the results. This appendix contains a summary of the findings of the survey.

The objectives

The aim of the survey was to answer the following questions:

- members' usage of alternative medicine practitioners
- reasons for use
- effect of treatment
- likelihood of using practitioners again
- likelihood of recommending to a friend
- satisfaction with treatment
- whether there was a cause to complain
- whether members paid for treatment.

Method

A questionnaire containing a number of questions on alternative medicine was sent to 20,000 *Which?* readers. The number of respondents at the cut-off date was 8,745, a response rate of 44 per cent.

Results

1 Have you ever used a practitioner of alternative (complementary) medicine?

Base: All respondents

Total	8,745
Yes	2,724 (31%)
No	5,719 (65%)
No reply	302 (3%)

Comments

Significantly more women than men answered yes to this question (40% *vs* 27%). The under-35s were the group least likely to have said yes (26% compared to 34% [35-64] and 29% [over 65]).

2 Which of the following practitioners have you consulted in the last 12 months?

Base: All respondents who have ever used complementary medicine

Total	2,724
Osteopath	28%
Chiropractor	17%
Homeopath	16%
Acupuncturist	12%
Aromatherapist	12%
Reflexologist	9%
Psychotherapist/counsellor	8%
Herbalist	6%
Faith/spiritual healer	5%
Hypnotherapist	4%
Alexander technique teacher	3%
Naturopath	2%
Other alternative medicine practitioner	5%
None: have not visited in last 12 months	23%
No reply	4%

Comments

Nearly eight out of ten users of alternative medicines had consulted their practitioner within the last 12 months. Of these, 1,078 (38%) had visited more than one type of practitioner and had on average visited 1.3 types of practitioner. The most popular type of practitioner among *Which?* readers are osteopaths (28%) and chiropractors (17%). Osteopaths are significantly more likely to be used by men (30% *vs* 25%) and the over-65s (36%). Women are significantly more likely to have used aromatherapists (18% *vs* 8%) or homeopaths (18% *vs* 14%). Aromatherapists are more likely to be used by younger age groups (18% under 35, 12% between 35 and 64, and 5% over-65).

3 **Did you see the practitioner as an NHS (non-paying) patient, or did you pay privately?**

Base: All those who stated which practitioner they had seen most often or most recently in the previous 12 months

Total	1,874
Private	85%
NHS	7%
No reply	8%

Comment

The majority of visits to alternative practitioners are, as expected, carried out privately. The practitioners who are most likely to be available on the NHS are psychotherapists/counsellors (27% of visits on the NHS) and acupuncturists (21% on the NHS).

4 **What was the reason for the last visit to an alternative practitioner?**

Base: All those who stated which practitioner they had seen most often or most recently in the previous 12 months

Total	1,874
New health problem	18%
Long-term health problem	41%
Ongoing consultation/not problem specific	11%
Dissatisfied with orthodox treatment	28%
Belief in approach of alternative medicine	34%
No reply	13%

Comments

The most likely reason for someone to visit an alternative practitioner is to deal with a long-term health problem. This is particularly so for chiropractors (48%) and faith/spiritual healers (48%). The therapists who attract the highest proportion of people who are dissatisfied with orthodox treatment are chiropractors (38%), homeopaths (34%), osteopaths (33%) and naturopaths (33%).

Over half the people who used aromatherapy, faith healing, naturopathy and reflexology stated that the reason for their last visit to a practitioner was because they believed in the general approach of alternative medicine: women were more likely than men to hold this view (43% *vs* 29%).

5 **Overall, has your condition improved, deteriorated or stayed the same as a direct result of this alternative treatment?**

Base: All those who stated which practitioner they had seen most often or most recently in the previous 12 months

Total	1,874
Improved greatly	46%
Improved slightly	28%
Stayed the same	12%
Deteriorated slightly	1%
Deteriorated greatly	<1%
Don't know/too soon to say	3%
No pre-existing condition	3%
No reply	7%

Comments

It is important to recognise that this is the respondents' view of their condition. Consumers' Association cannot affirm that these figures are an accurate indication of the performance of the therapies.

Three-quarters of users reported that their condition had improved to some degree after being treated by alternative practitioners. The therapies for which over half of the users reported that their condition had improved greatly were chiropractic (59%), osteopathy (58%) and faith/spiritual healing (52%). Only for hypnotherapy did fewer than 50% report an improvement.

Age or gender does not seem to have had any influence on users' perception of improvement.

6 Regardless of the outcome of the treatment, do you personally feel better, worse, or no different after visiting the alternative practitioner?

Base: All those who stated which practitioner they had seen most often or most recently in the previous 12 months

Total	1,874
Feel much better	54%
Feel slightly better	29%
Feel no different	15%
Feel slightly worse	1%
Feel much worse	<1%
No reply	<1%

Comment

The results here show an even more positive response than did the previous question on the level of improvement in the users' condition. Irrespective of the effect alternative medicine had on their condition, users tend to feel better in themselves after treatment. Even in the poorest performer, hypnotherapy, 58% of users felt better in themselves after treatment. Again, age or gender do not seem to affect the response to this question.

7 **Taking everything into consideration, how satisfied have you been with your complementary treatment?**

Base: All those who stated which practitioner they had seen most often or most recently in the previous 12 months

Total	1,874
Very satisfied	54%
Fairly satisfied	30%
Not very satisfied	7%
Not at all satisfied	2%
No reply	7%

Comment

A high level of satisfaction exists among the users of the various types of practitioner. Women are likely to be more satisfied than men; however, the difference is more to do with the degree of satisfaction rather than with more men being dissatisfied.

Therapies where there is a significantly high level of satisfaction are chiropractic (net 89% satisfied) and osteopathy (net 86% satisfied). Those therapies with a significantly lower level of satisfaction are herbalism (net 78% satisfied) and hypnotherapy (net 50% satisfied). The therapy that comes out worst overall is hypnotherapy, for which a net dissatisfaction among users of 41% is revealed, including 16% of users who were not at all satisfied.

8 **Would you recommend this alternative treatment to a relative or friend with the same problem?**

Base: All those who stated which practitioner they had seen most often or most recently in the previous 12 months

Total	1,874
Yes, definitely	57%
Yes, probably	22%
Don't know/not sure	7%
No, probably not	5%
No, definitely not	2%
No reply	7%

Comment

This is an clear endorsement from respondents for alternative medicine. Women are slightly more likely than men to recommend the therapy they used to a friend (60% *vs* 56%). The types of therapy that are most likely to be recommended are osteopathy (net yes 84%), aromatherapy (net yes 90%) and chiropractic (net yes 86%). Those that are less likely to be recommended are homeopathy (net yes 71%), herbalism (net yes 71%) and hypnotherapy (net yes 40%).

9 **Did you want to make a complaint about any aspect of this alternative treatment?**

Base: All those who stated which practitioner they had seen most often or most recently in the previous 12 months

Total	1,874
Yes	2%
No	90%
No reply	8%

Comment

This result mirrors the general level of satisfaction with alternative therapies.

Conclusions

People who are inclined to use alternative medicine are generally satisfied with the results. However, the 'satisfaction' results are based upon those who had used an alternative practitioner in the last 12 months. Of the 2,724 who had used an alternative practitioner in the past, 619 (23%) had not done so in the last 12 months. It could be the case that these people had not used a practitioner in the past 12 months because they were not satisfied with their previous experience.

The level of satisfaction appears to be correlated more to the feeling of general well-being resulting from treatment than from the effect it has on the condition for which patients initially saw the therapist.

Although these results cannot be used to make claims about the effectiveness of alternative medicine – full clinical trials would be necessary for that – they do show that the majority of people who use alternative medicines do benefit in some way.

GLOSSARY

Acupoints Points along the meridians (q.v.) which can be manipulated either by acupuncture or by pressure with the hands to bring about health and well-being

Aura An energy field said to be emitted by all living things. Some healers claim to see auras which take on different colours depending on the individual's state of health

Chakra A Sanskrit word meaning 'wheel'. In yogic philosophy the body has seven *chakras*, points along the spinal column through which life energy (*prana*) interacts with the body and mind

Endorphins Small morphine-like proteins which act as the body's natural painkillers. As well as dealing with pain, endorphins may control the body's response to stress. Acupuncture is thought to work partly by stimulating the release of endorphins

Immune system The body's defence system against invading bacteria and viruses and its own abnormal cells, such as cancer. In auto-immune diseases, such as rheumatoid arthritis, the body attacks its own normal cells. Some therapies are said to boost the immune system

Mantra From the Sanskrit word meaning 'instrument of thought': a word or phrase repeated during meditation to help focus the mind

Meridians In Chinese medicine, a network of invisible pathways in the body. Along them flows a life-energy or *qi* (*q.v.*). When these become unbalanced, blocked or 'stagnant', the individual falls ill. There are 12 main meridians, with 365 acupoints (*q.v.*) located on them

Moxibustion Derived from the Japanese word *moekusa*, meaning 'burning herb', and often used in acupuncture to warm the *qi* (*q.v.*). The practitioner places a small cone of the powdered leaves of a herb, usually mugwort, over an acupuncture point. The herb is then lit and allowed to smoulder until the heat becomes almost unbearable, then it is removed. This is repeated several times on the same point

Placebo From Latin 'I shall please'. A placebo may be a medicine which is given more to please than to benefit the patient, who believes that taking a medicine will help. The belief in the healing power of medicine plays an important part in the restoration of one's health: the action of taking the medicine adds to the effectiveness of the drug. This is known as the 'placebo effect' or 'placebo response'. The word 'placebo' is also used to describe a 'dummy drug', an inactive substance which has no pharmacological effect on the body and which is used in clinical trials to test the effects of a medicine

Prana Universal life energy believed to be associated with breathing and absorbed into the body via the *chakras*; similar to *qi* (*q.v.*)

Psychoneuroimmunology An area of orthodox medical research investigating the links between the mind and the body. Scientists say it is possible that how we feel can affect neurotransmitters, or brain chemicals, which carry messages to the immune system and nervous system. In other words, our emotions can affect our health

Qi (pronounced 'chee') In traditional Chinese medicine, the life force or vital energy which circulates between the organs along channels called meridians (*q.v.*)

Visualisation A technique of using the imagination to create an image of changes that you want to make to your life

Yin/yang The dynamic balance of energy in traditional Chinese medicine. *Yang* energy is characterised by heat, movement, light and energy, and *yin* by darkness, inactivity, sluggishness and deficiency. A healthy person has a balance of each kind of energy

Zones In reflexology the body is divided into zones by vertical lines which run from the feet up the body to the head and down to the hands. Energy currents flow along these lines and illness results if there is an energy blockage in any zone

ADDRESSES

General

Action for Victims of Medical
Accidents
Bank Chambers
1 London Road
Forest Hill
London SE23 3TP
0181-291 2793

British Complementary Medicine
Association
9 Soar Lane
Leicester LE3 5DE
0116-242 5406

British Holistic Medical Association
Roland Thomas House
Royal Shrewsbury Hospital South
Shrewsbury SY3 8XF
(01743) 261155

Council for Complementary and
Alternative Medicine
Park House
206–208 Latimer Road
London W10 6RE
0181-968 3862

Health Information Line: 0800
665544

HealthWatch
Box CAHF
London WC1N 3XX
(01483) 503106

Institute for Complementary
Medicine
PO Box 194
London SE16 1QZ
0171-237 5165

Law Society Accident Line: 0500
192939

Legal Aid Board
85 Gray's Inn Road
London WC1X 8AA
0171-813 1000

Medical Negligence Panel
Ipsley Court
Redditch B98 OTD
0171- 242 1222 ext 3315

Medicines Control Agency
1 Nine Elms Lane
London SW8 5NQ
0171-273 0000

Natural Medicines Society
Market Chambers
13a Market Place
Heanor DE75 7AA
(01773) 710002

The Research Council for
Complementary Medicine
60 Great Ormond Street
London WC1N 3JF
0171-833 8897

Acupuncture

British Acupuncture Council
Park House
206-208 Latimer Road
London W10 6RE
0181-964 0222

British Medical Acupuncture Society
Newton House
Newton Lane
Whitley
Warrington WA4 4JA
(01925) 730727
Internet:
http://users.aol.com/acubmas.bmas.html

Alexander technique

Society of Teachers of the Alexander
Technique
20 London House
266 Fulham Road
London SW10 9EL
0171-351 0828

Aromatherapy

Aromatherapy Organisations Council
3 Latymer Close
Braybrooke
Market Harborough LE16 8LN
(01858) 434242

Aromatherapy Trade Council
PO Box 52
Market Harborough
Leicester LE16 8ZX
(*Send an sae for a general information
booklet*)

Art therapies

Association for Dance Movement
Therapy
c/o The Art Therapies Department
Springfield Hospital
Glenburnie Road
London SW17 7DJ
(*Send an sae for a general information
booklet*)

Association of Drama Therapists
4 Funnydale Villas
Durlston Road
Swanage BN19 2HY

British Association of Art Therapists
11a Richmond Road
Brighton BN2 3RL

British Society for Music Therapy
25 Rosslyn Avenue
East Barnet EN4 8DH
0181-368 8879

Inner Sound
8 Elms Avenue
London N10 2JP
0181-444 4855
(*For sound healing*)

Ayurvedic medicine

Ayurvedic Company of Great Britain
50 Penywern Road
London SW5 9SX
0171-370 2255/6

Ayurvedic Medical Association UK
59 Dulverton Road
South Croydon CR2 8PJ
0181-657 6147

Maharishi Ayur-Veda Health Centre
The Golden Dome
Woodley Park
Skelmersdale WN8 6UQ
(01695) 51008

Chinese herbal medicine

Register of Chinese Herbal Medicine
PO Box 400
Wembley HA9 9NZ
0181-904 1357 (answerphone)

Chiropractic

British Association for Applied
Chiropractic (McTimoney-Corley)
The Old Post Office
Cherry Street
Stratton Audley
Nr. Bicester OX6 9BA
(01869) 277111

British Chiropractic Association
29 Whitley Street
Reading RG2 OEG
(01734) 757557

McTimoney Chiropractic
Association
21 High Street
Eynsham OX8 1HE
(01865) 880974

National Back Pain Association
16 Elmtree Road
Teddington TW11 8ST
0181-977 5474

Scottish Chiropractic Association
30 Roseburn Place
Edinburgh EH12 5NX
0131-346 7500

Colonic hydrotherapy

Colonic International Association
16 Englands Lane
London NW3 4TG
0171-483 1595

Colour therapy

International Association of Colour
Therapy
PO Box 3
Potters Bar EN6 3ET
(01707) 876928

Crystal and gem healing

Affiliation of Crystal Healing
Organisations
46 Lower Green Road
Esher KT10 8HD
0181-398 7252

Flower remedies

The Dr Edward Bach Centre
Mount Vernon
Bakers Lane
Sotwell
Wallingford OX10 0PZ
(01491) 834678

Healing

Confederation of Healing
Organisations
Suite J
113 High Street
Berkhamsted HP4 2DJ
(01442) 870660

National Federation of Spiritual
Healers
Old Manor Farm Studio
Church Street
Sunbury-on-Thames TW16 6RG
(01932) 783164

Herbal medicine

National Institute of Medical
Herbalists
56 Longbrook Street
Exeter EX4 6AH
(01392) 426022

Homeopathy

British Homoeopathic Association
27A Devonshire Street
London W1N 1RJ
0171-935 2163

Faculty of Homoeopathy
2 Powis Place
Great Ormond Street
London WCIN 3HT
0171-837 9469

Society of Homoeopaths
2 Artizan Road
Northampton NN1 4HU
(01604) 21400

Hypnotherapy

British Society of Experimental and
Clinical Hypnosis
% Dept of Psychology
Grimsby General Hospital
Scartho Road
Grimsby DN33 2BA
(01472) 879238

British Society of Medical and
Dental Hypnosis
17 Keppel View Road
Kimberworth
Rotherham S61 2AR
(01709) 554558

British Society of Medical and
Dental Hypnosis (Scotland)
PO Box 1007
Glasgow G31 2LE
0141-556 1606

National School of Hypnotherapy
and Psychotherapy
The Central Register of Advanced
Hypnotherapists
28 Finsbury Park Road
London N4 2JX
0171-359 6991

Iridology

Guild of Naturopathic Iridologists
94 Grosvenor Road
London SW1V 3LF
0171-834 3579

International Association of Clinical
Iridologists
853 Finchley Road
London NW1 8LX
0181-458 7781

Kinesiology

Association of Systematic
Kinesiology
39 Browns Road
Surbiton KT5 8ST
0181-399 3215

The Kinesiology Federation
PO Box 7891
London SW19 1ZB
0181-545 0255

Massage therapy

Bodyharmonics
54 Flecker's Drive
Hatherley
Cheltenham GL51 5DB
(01242) 582168
(*For* tuina *massage*)

British Massage Therapy Council
Greenbank House
65a Adelphi Street
Preston PR1 7BH
(01772) 881063

Hale Clinic
7 Park Crescent
London W1N 3HE
0171-631 0156
(*For* marma *and* tuina *massage*)

London School of Sports Massage
PO Box 46
Battle TN33 OZH
(01424) 870199

Massage Therapy Institute of Great
Britain
PO Box 2726
London NW2 4NR
0181-208 1607

Meditation

Friends of the Western Buddhist
Order
London Buddhist Centre
51 Roman Road
London E2 0HU
0181-981 1225

School of Meditation
158 Holland Park Avenue
London W11 4UH
0171-603 6116

Transcendental Meditation
Freepost
London SW1P 4YY
(0990) 143733

Metamorphic technique

Metamorphic Association
67 Ritherdon Road
London SW17 8QE
0181-672 5951
(*Send an sae for information*)

Naturopathy

General Council and Register of
Naturopaths
Goswell House
2 Goswell Road
Street BA16 0JG
(01458) 840072

Osteopathy

College of Osteopathic Practitioners
Association
13 Furzehill Road
Borehamwood
WD6 2DG
0181-905 1937

General Council and Register of
Osteopaths
56 London Street
Reading RG1 4SQ
(01734) 576585

Guild of Osteopaths
497 Bury New Road
Prestwich
Manchester M25 1AD
0161-798 6352

National Back Pain Association
(*see Chiropractic*)

Natural Therapeutic and
Osteopathic Society and Register
63 Collingwood Road
Witham CM8 2EE
(01376) 512188

Osteopathic Information Service
PO Box 2074
Reading RG1 4YR
(01734) 512051

Radiesthesia and radionics

Confederation of Radionics and
Radiesthesic Organisations
Radionics and Radiesthesia Trust
Wincanton BA9 8EH
(01963) 32651

Radionic Association
Baerlein House
Goose Green
Deddington
Banbury OX15 0SZ
(01869) 338852

Reflexology

Association of Reflexologists
27 Old Gloucester Street
London WC1 3XX
(0990) 673320

British Reflexology Association
Monks Orchard
Whitbourne
Worcester WR6 5RB
(01886) 821207

British School of Reflex Zone
Therapy of the Feet
23 Marsh Hall
Talisman Way
Wembley Park
London HA9 8JJ
0181-904 4825

Rolfing

Rolf Institute of Structural
Integration
PO Box 1868
Boulder
Colorado 80306
USA

UK contact: 0171-834 1493

Shiatsu

Shiatsu Society
31 Pullman Lane
Godalming GU7 1XY
(01483) 860771

T'ai chi

School of T'ai-chi Ch'uan Centre for
Healing
5 Tavistock Place
London WC1H 9SN
0181-444 6445

T'ai Chi Union for Great Britain
23 Oakwood Avenue
Mitcham CR4 3DQ

Yoga

British Wheel of Yoga
1 Hamilton Place
Boston Road
Sleaford NG34 7ES
(01529) 306851

Iyengar Yoga Institute
223a Randolph Avenue
London W9 1NL
0171-624 3080

Yoga Biomedical Trust
PO Box 140
Cambridge CB1 1U

Yoga for Health Foundation
Ickwell Bury
Ickwell Green
Biggleswade SG18 9EF
(01767) 627271

Yoga Therapy Centre
Royal London Homeopathic
Hospital Trust
60 Great Ormond Street
London WC1N 3HR
0171-833 7267

BIBLIOGRAPHY

General

Barrett, S., Jarvis, W.T. (ed) 1995. *Health robbers: a close look at quackery in America*. Prometheus

Benson, H. 1996. *Timeless healing: the power and biology of belief*. Simon & Schuster

Brown, L. 1994. *Working in complementary and alternative medicine*. Kogan Page

Coward, R. 1989. *The whole truth: the myth of alternative health*. Faber

Pantanowitz, D. 1995. *Alternative medicine: a doctor's perspective*. Southern Books

Sharma, U. 1991. *Complementary medicine today: practitioners and patients*. Routledge

Stalker, D., Glymour, C. (ed) 1986. *Examining holistic medicine*. Prometheus

Stanway, A. 1994. *Complementary medicine: a guide to natural therapies*. Penguin

Stanway, A. (ed) 1996. *The new natural family doctor*. Gaia

Vickers, A.J. 1993. *Complementary medicine and disability*. Chapman & Hall

Vickers, A.J. 1994. *Health options: complementary therapies for cerebral palsy and related conditions*. Element

Woodham, A. 1994. *HEA guide to complementary medicine and therapies*. Health Education Authority

Healthy choice. *Which?*, November 1995, pp 8-13

Risking the alternative. *Health Which?*, December 1995, pp 196-9

Chapter 1   Complementary therapies, their users and providers

Eisenberg, D. *et al*. 1993. Unconventional medicine in the United States – prevalence, costs and patterns of use. *New England Journal of Medicine*, **328**, 246-52

Chapter 2   Complementary medicine and the NHS

British Medical Association. 1986. *Alternative therapy*. Chameleon Press

British Medical Association. 1993. *Complementary medicine: new approaches to good practice*. Oxford University Press

Thomas, K. *et al.* 1995. *The national survey of access to complementary health care via general practice.* Medical Care Research Unit, University of Sheffield

Chapter 3   The scientific case for complementary medicine

[1] Vickers, A.J. 1996. Can acupuncture have specific effects on health? A systematic literature review of acupuncture antiemesis trials. *Journal of the Royal Society of Medicine,* **89,** 303-11

[2] Pomeranz, B. *et al.* 1974. Acupuncture reduces electrophysiological and behavioral responses to noxious stimuli: pituitary is implicated. *Experimental Neurology,* **54,** 172-8

[3] Saku, K. *et al.* 1993. Characteristics of reactive electropermeable points on the auricles of coronary heart disease patients. *Clinical Cardiology,* **16,** 415-19

[4] Kleijnen, J. *et al.* 1991. Clinical trials of homoeopathy. *British Medical Journal,* **302,** 316-23

[5] Meade, T.W. *et al.* 1990. Low back pain of mechanical origin: randomised comparison of chiropractic and hospital outpatient treatment. *British Medical Journal,* **300,** 1431-7

[6] Koes, B.W. *et al.* 1991. Spinal manipulation and mobilisation for back and neck pain: a blinded review. *British Medical Journal,* **303,**1298-303

[7] Koes, B.W. *et al.* 1992. Randomised clinical trial of manipulative therapy and physiotherapy for persistent back and neck complaints: results of one-year follow-up. *British Medical Journal,* **304,** 601-5

[8] Meade, T.W. *et al.* 1995. Randomised comparison of chiropractic and ·hospital outpatient management for low back pain: results from extended follow-up. *British Medical Journal,* **311,** 349-51

[9] Nielsen, N.H. *et al.* 1995. Chronic asthma and chiropractic spinal manipulation: a randomized clinical trial. *Clinical & Experimental Allergy,* **25,** 80-8

[10] Morgan, J.P. 1985. A controlled trial of spinal manipulation in the management of hypertension. *Journal of the American Osteopathic Association,* **85,** 308-13

[11] Fischer-Rasmussen, W. *et al.* 1991. Ginger treatment of hyperemesis gravidarum. *European Journal of Obstetrics, Gynaecology & Reproductive Biology,* **38,** 19-24

[12] Linde, K. *et al.* 1996. St John's wort for depression – an overview and meta-analysis of randomised clinical trials. *British Medical Journal,* **313,** 253-8

[13] Ewer, T.C., Stewart, D.E. 1986. Improvement in bronchial hyper-responsiveness in patients with moderate asthma after treatment with a hypnotic technique: a randomised controlled trial. *British Medical Journal,* **293,** 1129-32

[14] Whorwell, P.J. *et al.* 1984. Controlled trial of hypnotherapy in the treatment of severe refractory irritable bowel syndrome. *Lancet,* **2,** 1232-4

[15] Melis, P.M. *et al.* 1991. Treatment of chronic tension-type headache with hypnotherapy: a single-blind time-controlled study. *Headache,* **31,** 686-9

[16] Lambe, R. *et al*. 1986. A randomized controlled trial of hypnotherapy for smoking cessation. *Journal of Family Practice*, **22**, 61-5

[17] Panusch, R.S., 1983. Diet therapy for rheumatoid arthritis. *Arthritis and Rheumatism*, **26**, 462-8

[18] Darlington, L.G. *et al*. 1986. Placebo-controlled, blind study of dietary manipulation therapy in rheumatoid arthritis. *Lancet*, **1**, 236-8

[19] Egger, J. *et al*. 1983. Is migraine food allergy?: A double-blind controlled trial of oligoantigenic diet treatment. *Lancet*, **2**, 865-9

[20] Egger, J. 1985. A controlled trial of oligoantigenic diet treatment in the hyperkinetic syndrome. *Lancet*, **1**, 540-5

[21] Field, T. *et al*. 1992. Massage reduces anxiety in child and adolescent psychiatric patients. *Journal of American Academy of Child and Adolescent Psychology*, **31**, 125-31

[22] Stevensen, C. 1994. The psychophysiological effects of aromatherapy massage following cardiac surgery. *Complementary Therapies in Medicine,* **2**, 27-35

[23] Bassett, I.B. *et al*. 1990. A comparative study of tea-tree oil *versus* benzoylperoxide in the treatment of acne. *Medical Journal of Australia*, **153**, 455-8

[24] Tong, M.M. *et al*. 1992. Tea-tree oil in the treatment of tinea pedis. *Australasian Journal of Dermatology*, **33**, 145-9

[25] Sethi, T.J. *et al*. 1987. How reliable are commercial allergy tests? *Lancet*, **10**, 92-4

[26] Barret, S. 1985. Commercial hair analysis: science or scam? *Journal of the American Medical Association,* **254**, 1041-3

[27] Knipschild, P. 1988. Looking for gall bladder disease in the patient's iris. *British Medical Journal*, **297**, 1578-81

[28] Simon, A. *et al*. 1979. An evaluation of iridology. *Journal of the American Medical Association*, **242**, 1385-9

[29] Kenney, J.J. *et al*. 1988. Applied kinesiology: unreliable for assessing nutrient status. *Journal of the American Diet Association*, **88**, 698-704

Chapter 4 Complementary medicine: the good, the bad and the unknown

Gill, G.V. *et al*. 1994. Diabetes and alternative medicine: cause for concern. *Diabetic Medicine*, **11**, 210-13

Sims, S. 1988. The significance of touch in palliative care. *Palliative Medicine*, **2**, 58-61

Spiegel, D. *et al*. 1989. Effect of psychosocial treatment on survival of patients with metastatic breast cancer. *Lancet*, **2**, 888-91

Chapter 5 Complementary medicine and the law

Medawar, C. *et al*. (ed) 1992. *Power and dependence: social audit on the safety of medicines*. Social Audit Ltd

Stone, J., Matthews, J. 1996. *Complementary medicine and the law*. Oxford University Press

Acupuncture

Christensen, B.V. *et al.* 1992. Acupuncture treatment of severe knee osteoarthritis. *Acta Anaesthesiologica Scandinavica*, **36**, 519-25

Jobst, K. 1996. Acupuncture in asthma and pulmonary diseases: an analysis of efficacy and safety. *Journal of Alternative and Complementary Medicine*, **2**, 179-206

Mole, P. 1992. *Acupuncture: energy balancing for body, mind and spirit*. Element

Nightingale, M. 1992. *Acupuncture*. Optima

Norheim, A. J., Fønnebø, V. 1996. Acupuncture: adverse effects are more than occasional: case reports. *Complementary Therapies in Medicine*, **14**, 8-13

Rampes, H., James, R. 1995. Complications in acupuncture. *Acupuncture in Medicine*, **13**, 26-34

Vickers, A.J. 1996. Can acupuncture have specific effects on health? A systematic literature review of acupuncture antiemesis trials. *Journal of the Royal Society of Medicine*, **89**, 303-11

Alexander technique

Hodgkinson, L. 1988. *The Alexander technique*. Piatkus

Stevens, C. 1996. *Alexander technique: an introductory guide to the technique and its benefits*. Vermilion

Aromatherapy

Dunn, C. *et al.* 1995. Sensing an improvement: an experimental study to evaluate the use of aromatherapy, massage and periods of rest in an intensive care unit. *Journal of Advanced Nursing*, **21**, 34-40

Stevensen, C. 1994. The psychophysiological effects of aromatherapy massage following cardiac surgery. *Complementary Therapies in Medicine*, **2**, 27-35

Tisserand, R. 1977. *The art of aromatherapy*. C. W. Daniel

Tisserand, R. 1990. *Aromatherapy for everyone*. Penguin

Tisserand, R. 1995. *Essential oil safety: a guide for health care*. Churchill Livingstone

Van Toller, S., Dodd, G. H. (ed) 1993. *Fragrance: the psychology and biology of perfume*. Elsevier

Art therapies

Bunt, L. 1994. *Music therapy: an art beyond words*. Routledge

Case, C., Dalley, T. (ed) 1990. *Working with children in art therapy*. Routledge

Ayurveda

Aslam, M. *et al.* 1979. Heavy metals in some Asian medicines and cosmetics. *Public Health*, **93**, 274-84

Donal, G. *et al.* 1991. Lead poisoning due to Asian ethnic treatment for impotence. *Journal of the Royal Society of Medicine*, **84**, 630-1

Chinese herbal medicine

De Smet, P.A.G.M. 1995. Health risks of herbal remedies. *Drug Safety*, **13**, 81-3
Kaptchuk, T.J. 1987. *Chinese medicine: the web that has no weaver*. Century
Shaw, D. *et al*. 1996. *Toxicological problems resulting from exposure to traditional medicines and food supplements*. Medical Toxicology Unit, Guy's & St Thomas' Hospital Trust
Tiquia, R. 1996. *Traditional Chinese medicine*. Australian Consumers' Association
Xu, G. 1996. *Chinese herbal medicine*. Vermilion

Chiropractic

Carrington, M., Breen, A. 1996. Chiropractic, osteopathy and physiotherapy: general practitioners' perceptions on their roles in the treatment of low back pain. *Proceedings of the Seventh International Conference on Spinal Manipulation*, Bournemouth
Lee, K. P. *et al*. 1995. Neurologic complications following chiropractic manipulation: a survey of Californian neurologists. *Neurology*, **45**, 1213-15
Moore, J.S. 1993. *Chiropractic in America*. Johns Hopkins University Press

Colour therapy

Bonds, L.V., Gimbel, T. 1993. *The colour therapy workbook*. Element
Bonds, L.V. 1994. *Discover the magic of colour*. Optima
Wills, P. 1992. *The reflexology and colour therapy workbook*. Element

Flower remedies

Mansfield, P. 1995. *Flower remedies*. Optima

Healing

Benor, D. J., Netzer, N. (ed) 1993. *Healing research: holistic energy medicine and spirituality*. Helix Books
Buckman, R., Sabbagh, K. 1994. *Magic or medicine? An investigation into healing*. Pan

Herbal medicine

Linde, K. *et al*. 1996. St John's wort for depression – an overview and meta-analysis of randomised clinical trials. *British Medical Journal*, **313**, 253-8
Mills, S. 1994. *The complete guide to modern herbalism*. Thorsons
Shaw, D. *et al*. 1996. *Toxicological problems resulting from exposure to traditional medicines and food supplements*. Medical Toxicology Unit, Guy's & St Thomas' Hospital Trust

Homeopathy

Kleijnen, J. *et al*. 1991. Clinical trials of homeopathy. *British Medical Journal*, **302**, 316-23
Reilly, D., Taylor, M. 1985. Potent placebo or potency? A proposed study model with initial findings using homoeopathy prepared pollens in hay fever. *British Homeoepathic Journal*, **74**, 65

Homeopathy off the shelf. *Which? Way to Health*, October 1992, pp 158-60

Hypnotherapy

Jenkins, M.W., Pritchard, M. 1993. Hypnosis: practical applications and theoretical considerations in normal labour. *British Journal of Obstetrics and Gynaecology*, **100**, 221-6

Karle, H.W.A. 1988. *Hypnosis and hypnotherapy*. Thorsons

Stewart, A.C., Thomas, S.E. 1995. Hypnotherapy as a treatment for atopic dermatitis in adults and children. *British Journal of Dermatology*, **132**, 778-83

Whorwell, P. J. *et al*. 1984. Controlled trial of hypnotherapy in the treatment of severe refractory irritable bowel syndrome. *Lancet*, **2**, 1232-4

Iridology

Jackson, A. 1986. *Iridology: a practical guide to iris analysis*. Vermilion

Knipschild, P. 1988. Looking for gall bladder disease in the patient's iris. *British Medical Journal*, **297**, 1578-81

Simon, A. *et al*. 1979. An evaluation of iridology. *Journal of the American Medical Association*, **242**, 1385-9

Kinesiology

Butler, B. (ed) *et al*. 1992. *Kinesiology for balanced health*. TASK

Butler, B. 1995. *An introduction to kinesiology*. TASK

Courtenay, A., la Tourelle, M. 1992. *Thorsons introductory guide to kinesiology*. Thorsons

Garrow, J.S. 1988. Kinesiology and food allergy. *British Medical Journal*, **296**, 1573-4

Haas, M. *et al*. 1994. Muscle testing response to provocative vertebral challenge and spinal manipulation: a randomized controlled trial of construct validity. *Journal of Manipulative & Physiological Therapeutics*, **17**, 141-8

Kenney, J.J. *et al*. 1988. Applied kinesiology: unreliable for assessing nutrient status. *Journal of the American Diet Association*, **88**, 698-704

Massage

Corner J. *et al*. 1995. An evaluation of the use of massage and essential oils on the wellbeing of cancer patients. *International Journal of Palliative Nursing*, **1**, 67-73

Field, T. *et al*. 1986. Tactile/kinesthetic stimulation effects on preterm neonates. *Pediatrics*, **77**, 654-8

Field, T. *et al*. 1992. Massage reduces anxiety in child and adolescent psychiatric patients. *Journal of American Academy of Child and Adolescent Psychology*, **31**, 125-31

Stevensen, C. 1994. The psychophysiological effects of aromatherapy massage following cardiac surgery. *Complementary Therapies in Medicine*, **2**, 27-35

Vickers, A.J. 1996. *Massage and aromatherapy: a guide for health professionals*. Chapman & Hall

Meditation

Fontana, D. 1992. *The meditator's handbook*. Element
West, M. A. (ed) 1987. *The psychology of meditation*. Oxford University Press
Whiting, F. W. 1985. *Being oneself: the way of meditation*. School of Meditation
Zinn, J.K. 1996. *Full catastrophe living*. Piatkus

Metamorphic technique

Saint-Pierre, G., Shapiro, D.B. 1988. *The metamorphic technique: principles and practice*. Element

Naturopathy

Kjeldsen-Kragh J. *et al*. 1991. Controlled trial of fasting and one-year vegetarian diet in rheumatoid arthritis. *Lancet*, **338**, 899-902
Stampfer, M. J. *et al*. 1993. Vitamin E consumption and the risk of coronary disease in women. *New England Journal of Medicine*, **328**, 1444-9

Osteopathy

Koes, B.W. *et al*. 1991. Spinal manipulation and mobilisation for back and neck pain: a blinded review. *British Medical Journal*, **303**, 1298-303
Royal College of General Practitioners. 1996. *Clinical guidelines for the management of acute low back pain*.
Shekelle, P. *et al*. 1992. Spinal manipulation for low-back pain. *Annals of Internal Medicine*, **117**, 590-8
Szmelskyj, A. 1992. The qualifications and geographical distribution of practising osteopaths in England, Scotland and Wales. *Complementary Medical Research*, **6**, 1-8
Osteopathy. *Which? Way to Health*, October 1993, pp 173-5

Radiesthesia and radionics

Ernst, E., Hentschel, C. 1995. Diagnostic methods in complementary medicine. Which craft is witchcraft? *International Journal of Risk & Safety in Medicine*, **7**, 55-63
Russell, E.W. 1974. *Report on radionics*. Spearman

Reflexology

Oleson, T., Flocco, W. 1993. Randomised controlled study of premenstrual symptoms treated with ear, hand and foot reflexology. *Obstetrics and Gynaecology*, **82**, 906-11

Rolfing

Cottingham, J. *et al*. 1988. Shifts in pelvic inclination angle and parasympathetic tone produced by rolfing soft tissue manipulation. *Physical Therapy*, **68**, 1364-70

T'ai chi

Lai J.S. *et al.* 1995. Two-year trends in cardiorespiratory function among older Tai'chi chuan practitioners and sedentary subjects. *Journal of American Geriatrics Society*, **43**, 1222-7

Lan C. *et al.* 1996. Cardiorespiratory function, flexibility, and body composition among geriatric T'ai chi chuan practitioners. *Archives of Physical Medicine and Rehabilitation,* **77**, 612-16

Yoga

Monro, R. *et al.* 1992. Yoga therapy for NIDDM. *Complementary Medical Research*, **6**, 66-8

Nagarathna R., Nagendra R. 1985. Yoga for bronchial asthma: a controlled study. *British Medical Journal*, **291**, 1077-9

INDEX

absent/distant healing 137, 139
acne 33, 88, 102
Action for Victims of Medical Accidents
    61-2
acupressure 71, 78
acupuncture 8, 14, 17, 19, 27, 31, 40, 45,
    50, 52, 53, 54, 67, 71-81
addictions 75, 99, 163, 194, 227
aesthetic aromatherapy 88
alcohol dependence 99, 188
Alexander, Frederick Matthias 83
Alexander technique 8, 17, 82-6
allergic rhinitis 106
allergies 177-8, 198, 200, 211
allergy clinics 34
alternative medicine 7, 8
    see also complementary medicine
angina 162
animals 31, 90, 116, 133, 157, 211
anorexia 99, 162
anxiety 33, 75, 91, 96, 98, 99, 176, 184,
    185, 188, 190, 223
aphrodisiacs 104
aromatherapy 8, 17, 18, 26, 27, 33, 42, 46,
    87-95
art therapies 96-100
art therapy 96-7, 99-100
arteries, hardening of 170, 172
arthritis 14, 27, 33, 75, 83, 91, 102, 125,
    126, 140, 145, 147, 162, 200
asthma 32, 79, 106, 114, 125, 126, 127,
    147, 154, 159, 162, 163, 165, 182,
    198, 200, 206, 211, 216, 234, 327
astrology 101
athlete's foot 33
auras 124-5, 126, 136
autism 99, 126
ayurvedic medicine 19, 101-4

Bach, Edward 133
Bach flower remedies 46, 132

back pain 26, 47-8, 75, 83, 114, 116-17,
    118, 181, 182, 183, 185, 205-6,
    207-8, 216, 223, 226, 233-4, 237
bacterial infections 91
Bayley, Doreen 219
bedwetting 163
biokinesiology 178
bladder problems 215
bloating 120
blood pressure, high 33, 75, 93, 125, 127,
    145, 147, 150, 172, 190, 216, 232,
    237
bones, broken 137
bowel disorders 43, 120
    see also constipation; irritable bowel
        syndrome
Braid, James 163
Braunschweig, Heironymus 89
breast cancer 27, 37
breathing awareness 27
British Complementary Medicine
    Association 51, 57, 59
British Medical Association 8, 25, 86,
    138, 204
bronchitis 106, 234
Buddhist meditation 187, 188, 190-1, 192
bulimia 99

cancer 8, 27, 37, 38, 45-6, 125, 126, 137,
    147, 150, 185, 194, 202, 220, 227
chakras 40, 235
Chinese herbal medicine 8, 17, 18, 19,
    40, 105-12, 107
chiropractic 8, 14, 17, 32, 47-8, 53,
    113-19
Chiropractors Act 1994 50, 113
circulation, improving 121, 184, 216
clinical aromatherapy 88
colds and 'flu 14, 145, 147, 201, 234
colic 206
colonic hydrotherapy 8, 42, 120-3

colonic irrigation *see* colonic
      hydrotherapy
colour therapy 8, 124-8
complaints 57-68
      'consent' in medical practice 64-5
      legal action 59, 60-8
      procedures 57-60
complementary medicine
      advantages 35-8
      deciding to opt for 18-19
      discontinuing treatment 23
      'does it work?' 30-1
      drawbacks and criticisms of 38-40, 49
      finding a practitioner 19-23
      government attitude towards 52-3
      growth in popularity 7, 13-15
      holistic approach 15, 35-6
      mind-body link 37
      misconceptions 44-5
      not a substitute for conventional
            medicine 39-40
      outside the UK 15-16, 53-4
      patient involvement 15, 37-8
      patients' experiences 45-8
      randomised controlled trials (RCTs)
            29-30
      regulation 49-68
      safety 44
      scientific studies 29-34, 79, 90-2,
            116-17, 149, 157, 207-8
      term explained 8
      theories of the body 40-4
      users 16-17
complementary therapies
      aims and methods of practice 18
      combining 19
      range and diversity 8, 17-18
'consciousness widening' 98
'consent', principle of 64-5
constipation 43, 114, 120, 122, 159, 182,
      198, 206, 216, 220, 223
Council for Complementary and
      Alternative Medicine 52
counselling 9
cranial osteopathy 46, 205, 206
crystal and gem healing 8, 129-31
Culpeper, Nicholas 146
cupping 78
cystitis 75

dance movement therapy 98-9
de Morant, Georges Soulie 76
deaf and blind people 99
dementia 27, 92
depression 27, 32, 75, 83, 91, 96, 98, 99,
      121, 125, 127, 130, 140, 147-8, 166,
      176, 184, 185, 188, 190
detoxification 75, 103, 201
diabetes 39-40, 42, 93, 150, 172, 221, 237

diarrhoea 120
digestive problems 75, 88, 102, 106, 145,
      176, 182, 211, 234
diphtheria 147
'Dong diet' 33
Dorrell, Stephen 25
dowsing, medical *see* radiesthesia and
      radionics
drama therapy 99, 100
drug dependence 99, 188
dysentery 129

eating disorders 99, 162
eczema 19, 88, 102, 105, 108, 145, 154,
      164, 198, 216
Edwards, Harry 138
elderly people 8, 27, 92, 100, 181, 232
electro-acupuncture 76, 78
elimination diets 33, 46, 200, 202
endorphins 75, 184
enemas 121
energy 40-2, 136, 139-40, 182
      blocked and unblocked 18, 40, 72,
            175, 226
      channels 18, 216
      electromagnetic energy 41
      physical energy 41
      subtle energy 42
'entrained', becoming 41
epilepsy 92, 93, 127, 129, 150
essential oils *see* aromatherapy
eye disorders 129, 172, 202

faith healing 137
fasting 43, 200, 202
fatigue 14, 102
flatulence 120
flower remedies 8, 17, 132-5
folk medicine 9
food sensitivity 33, 177-8
free radicals 147, 201, 202
frozen shoulder 182

gall bladder disease 173
Gattefosse, René-Maurice 89
General Medical Council 50-1, 55
Gimbel, Theo 127
ginseng 147
glaucoma 172
glue ear 206
Goodheart, Dr George 176
gout 102
GPs
      consulting and liaising with 19, 20
      misconduct 50-1
      provision of complementary therapies
            25, 153

Hahnemann, Samuel 154-5
hay fever 75, 154, 159, 198, 200, 211, 234

headaches 26, 32, 43, 114, 121, 140, 176, 181, 190, 206, 216
healing 17, 46, 136-43
heart conditions 43, 127, 147, 185, 201, 202, 232, 237
hepatitis 106
herbal medicine 8, 13, 16, 17, 19, 32, 46, 52, 53, 54, 56, 101, 103, 144-51
  see also Chinese herbal medicine
Herbalists' Charter 55
HIV and AIDS 75, 99, 126, 127, 185, 227
holistic aromatherapy 88
homeopathy 8, 13, 16, 17, 19, 24, 27, 32, 46, 50, 52, 53, 54, 56, 152-60
humours (ayurvedic medicine) 102
hydrotherapy 198-9, 200
hyperacidity 170
hyperactivity 33
hypertension 32
hypnotherapy 17, 33, 37, 161-8

illness, mental attitudes to 39
immune system, boosting 37, 125, 147
impotence 102
indigestion 102
infertility 102
insomnia 27, 75, 91, 125, 148, 182, 188, 190, 220
Institute for Complementary Medicine 51-2, 57, 59, 128, 173
iridology 17, 18, 19, 34, 42, 43, 169-74, 200
irritable bowel syndrome (IBS) 14, 32, 75, 102, 114, 120, 121, 137, 145, 147, 154, 162, 165-6, 182, 188, 190, 198, 216, 234
Iskador therapy 27, 147

Jackson, Adam 173-5
joint problems 75, 102, 114, 145

ketoacidosis 40
kidneys, weak 170
kinesiology 17, 18, 34, 175-9
Knipschild, P 173

Laban, Rudolph 98
Lane, Sir William Arbuthnot 43
Lannoye, Paul 53
laxatives 120
laying-on of hands 17, 27, 137
  see also spiritual healing
learning difficulties 96, 99
Lewisham Hospital 26
Liebault, Ambroise 163
life force see ojas; prana; qi
limbic system 90, 91
Ling, Per Henrik 182
litigation 60-4
liver damage 110, 149
loss and bereavement 37, 99

Luo, Dr 108

manipulative and structural therapies 17
mantra meditation 188
marma massage 180-1, 182, 183
massage 8, 17, 19, 21, 26, 27, 33, 42, 46, 47, 90, 103, 180-6
McTimoney-Corley chiropractic 114, 116
Medical Act 1858 24, 55-6
Medical Negligence Panel 61
medicinal therapies 17
Medicines Act 1968 56-7, 109, 148
Medicines Control Agency 44, 109, 148
medicines and preparations
  licensing 44, 56-7, 109, 148-9
  product liability 67
meditation 17, 37, 101, 103, 141, 187-92, 235
melodic intonation 97-8
meningitis 147
menopausal problems 75, 88, 102
menstrual problems 75, 102, 106, 145
mental disabilities 8, 96, 99, 137
mental illness 96, 97, 98, 99, 194
meridians 29, 40, 72, 175, 226
Mesmer, Franz 163
metamorphic technique 17, 193-6
methicillin-resistant Staphylococcus aureus (MRSA) 91
middle ear problems 206
migraine 26, 33, 47-8, 75, 83, 102, 114, 126, 137, 148, 154, 168, 182, 188, 190, 198, 216
mind-body medicine 17
miscarriage 149
Moore, Alexander 45-7
morning sickness 32
moxibustion 78
multiple sclerosis 162, 231
muscle tension 83, 85, 162, 181, 222, 226
muscular aches and pains 88
musculo-skeletal problems 26, 83, 198, 205, 211, 223, 224, 226, 228
music therapy 97-8, 99, 100
myalgic encephalomyelitis (ME) 106, 121, 140, 194, 198

natural healing centres 20
Natural Medicines Society 52
naturopathy 42, 52, 197-203
nausea 31, 71, 75, 79, 220
neck pain 114, 182, 226
needle phobia 220
NHS and complementary medicine 14, 24-8
  care of the elderly 27
  changing attitudes 24-5
  complaints procedure 57, 60
  complementary therapies in hospitals 24, 26-7

training modules and courses 25
see also GPs
nutritional therapies 33, 46, 101, 103, 200, 202

obsessions 163
obsessive compulsive disorder 162
ojas (life force) 101
Oriental massage 181, 183
Oriental medicine 17, 71-2, 78
orthodox medicine, disillusionment with 7, 14, 18
osteoarthritis 206
Osteopaths Act 1993 50, 204
osteopathy 8, 14, 17, 18, 21, 32, 52, 53, 204-9
osteoporosis 117, 208, 229

pain relief 27, 33, 71, 75, 79, 85, 87, 97, 148, 162, 163, 166, 184, 185, 220
Palmer, David Daniel 114
panic attacks 163
period pains 88, 223
personality disorders 166
phlebitis 185
phobias 163, 168, 176
physical disabilities 8, 96, 99, 137, 227, 231, 234
phytotherapy *see* herbal medicine
placebo response 31, 32, 134, 140, 141, 157
pneumothorax 79
polarity reflex analysis 178
post-natal depression 190
postural problems 82, 114
postural techniques 17, 82-6, 222-5
practitioners 8, 19-23
    bad practitioners 22
    choosing 19-22
    complaints, making 57-68
    initial sessions 36
    legal action against 59, 60-8
    negligence 60, 61, 65-6
    professional organisations 20-1, 50
    questions to ask 21
    umbrella organisations 51-2
prana 40, 234-5
prayer 141
pregnancy 93, 114, 150, 158, 166, 185, 206, 208, 221, 229
premature ejaculation 102
premenstrual syndrome 88, 102, 106, 154, 188, 198, 206, 220
psoriasis 102, 140, 145, 216
psychiatric problems 98
psychic surgery 46
psychoneuroimmunology 37, 164
psychosis 99

qi 40, 72, 77, 105, 106, 226, 230

Quin, Dr Frederick 155

radiesthesia and radionics 17, 210-14
reflex zone therapy *see* reflexology
reflexology 8, 17, 26, 27, 215-21
regulation 49-68
    in Europe 53-4
    self-regulation 50, 51-2, 53
    state regulation 50, 54-7
reiki 8, 27, 137, 181, 182
relaxation 27, 37, 90, 92, 125, 162, 184, 187
repetitive strain injury 83, 140, 181
Rescue Remedy 133, 135
Research Council for Complementary Medicine 184-5
respiratory function, improving 85
respiratory problems 26, 75, 91, 145, 234
rheumatism 102, 154, 162
rheumatoid arthritis 14, 33, 43, 200, 206, 208
Rolf, Dr Ida 223
rolfing 8, 17, 222-5
rosacea 88
Royal London Homoeopathic Hospital 24, 27, 152, 155

Saint-Pierre, Gaston 194, 195, 196
schizophrenia 99, 166
sciatica 182, 185
self-help therapies 17
self-hypnosis 161
senile dementia 91
sexual problems 102
shiatsu 27, 226-9
sinusitis 75, 198, 206, 234
skin conditions 26, 88, 102, 106, 108, 145, 159, 216
sleeplessness *see* insomnia
smoking, giving up 32, 168
social phobias 163, 168
sore throats 145
sound therapy/sound healing 8, 98, 100
spinal manipulation 32, 117, 207-8
spiritual healing 137, 138
sports injuries 114
sprains 182
stage fright 83, 120
stammering and blushing 163
Still, Andrew Taylor 206
stomach ulcers 102, 145, 159, 234
stress 37, 75, 87, 125, 176, 183, 211, 219, 223, 226, 228, 237
stress-related conditions 83, 88, 140, 145, 154, 162, 180-1, 182, 188, 190, 195, 216
stretch marks 88
strokes 98, 117, 185
Swedish/Western massage 180-1, 182, 183, 184

t'ai chi 17, 18, 45, 230-2
Thai massage 180-1
thalamic pain 228-9
therapeutic touch 137
thrombosis 185
thyroid disorders 149, 221
'time lines' 193
tinnitus 147
Tisserand, Robert 89
tonics 104
total health 38-9
touch, healing power of 36
touch therapies 8, 17
toxins 42-3, 93, 120, 122, 199, 201, 202
transcendental meditation (TM) 187, 188, 189-90, 191
tuberculosis 147

tuina massage 181, 182
Turner, Christopher 47, 48
typhoid 147

ulcers 145, 149, 159, 234

varicose veins 185
vegetarianism 43
Vickers, Andrew 184-5
von Peczely, Ignatz 170, 172

Warner, Eugenie 47-8
weight reduction 121, 200
whiplash injuries 83, 183
wounds, healing 148

yin and *yang* 72, 105, 107, 230
yoga 17, 18, 19, 40, 101, 103, 233-8

READER'S REPORT FORM

If you cannot photocopy this form, please copy it out by hand or, better still, type it up, using the same structure. Fill it in as clearly as possible and send to: Dept NR, Freepost, Which? Ltd, 2 Marylebone Road, London NW1 1YN.

1. Have you ever used a complementary therapy?

    Yes ....
    No ....

2. Which of the following therapies have you used in the last 12 months?

1 Acupuncture ....
2 Alexander technique ....
3 Aromatherapy ....
4 Art therapies ....
5 Ayurvedic medicine ....
6 Chinese herbal medicine ....
7 Chiropractic ....
8 Colonic hydrotherapy ....
9 Colour therapy ....
10 Crystal & gem healing ....
11 Flower remedies ....
12 Healing ....
13 Herbal medicine ....
14 Homeopathy ....
15 Hypnotherapy ....
16 Iridology ....
17 Kinesiology ....
18 Massage therapy ....
19 Meditation ....
20 Metamorphic technique ....
21 Naturopathy ....
22 Osteopathy ....
23 Radiesthesia & radionics ....
24 Reflexology ....
25 Rolfing ....
26 Shiatsu ....
27 T'ai chi ....
28 Yoga ....
29 Other ....

Please answer questions 3 to 10 for those complementary therapists (up to three) you have visited most in the last 12 months. Please ensure that you answer all the questions for the same therapies and in the same order (e.g. if you used, say, acupuncture, meditation and yoga in the last 12 months, list them in the same order for each question, so acupuncture is always first, meditation second and yoga third). Please write the number of the therapy from the list above at the top of each column.

3. Did you see the therapist as an NHS (non-paying) patient or did you attend privately?

	Therapy (..........)	Therapy (...........)	Therapy (..........)
NHS			
Private			

4. Why did you visit a complementary therapist in the last 12 months?

	Therapy (..........)	Therapy (...........)	Therapy (..........)
New health problem			
Long-term health problem			
Not problem-specific			
Dissatisfaction with orthodox medicine			
Belief in general approach of therapy			
Other			

5. Overall, has your condition improved, deteriorated or stayed the same as a direct result of complementary therapy?

	Therapy (..........)	Therapy (...........)	Therapy (..........)
Improved greatly			
Improved slightly			
Stayed the same			
Deteriorated slightly			
Deteriorated greatly			
Don't know			
No pre-existing condition			

6. Regardless of the outcome of the treatment, do you personally feel much better, worse, or no different after visiting the practitioner?

	Therapy (..........)	Therapy (..........)	Therapy (..........)
Feel much better			
Feel slightly better			
Feel no different			
Feel slightly worse			
Feel much worse			

7. Taking everything into consideration, how satisfied have you been with the complementary therapies you have used?

	Therapy (..........)	Therapy (..........)	Therapy (..........)
Very satisfied			
Fairly satisfied			
Not very satisfied			
Not at all satisfied			

8. Would you recommend the therapies you have used to a relative or friend?

	Therapy (..........)	Therapy (..........)	Therapy (..........)
Yes, definitely			
Yes, probably			
Don't know/not sure			
No, probably not			
No, definitely not			

9. Did you make a complaint (or wish to) about any aspect of the therapies you used?

	Therapy (..........)	Therapy (..........)	Therapy (..........)
Yes			
No			

10. Please give details of what you wanted to complain about, why, whether you complained, to whom and with what result.

Personal details

Age: Under 35 ......   35-65 ......   Over 65 ......
Sex: Male ......   Female ......
Town/city ....   Postcode ....
Date ....

Please note that the results from the survey will be used in aggregated form only and your confidentiality will be assured.

Any comments